Y0-AEX-723

Author: Dr. Vickie Salter, PhD, MSN, RN

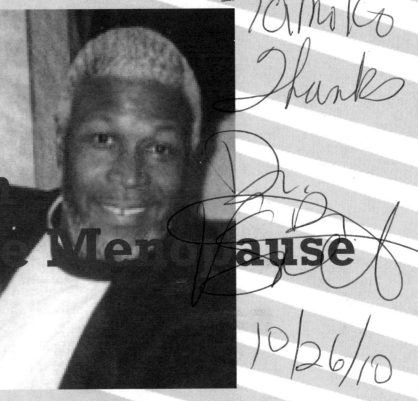

The Man, Male Menopause

Tamiko
Thanks

10/26/10

and
The Lost Libido

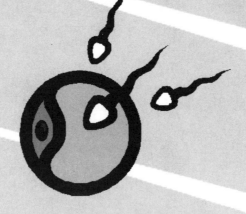

BASED ON RESEARCH!

Published in 2006 by: Dr. Vickie Salter, PhD, MSN, RN

Dr. Vickie Salter, PhD, MSN, RN
Email: drvickie@gmail.com
*Available for speaking engagements and seminars

Copyright © 2006 by Dr. Vickie Salter, PhD, MSN, RN
All rights reserved

Printed in the United States of America
MAYS PRINTING COMPANY, Inc.
15800 Livernois Avenue • Detroit, Michigan 48238
313.861.1900 • A Certified Minority Printer
www.maysprinting.com

No Part of this book amy be reprinted or reproduced or utilized in any form or by any electronic, mechanical or other means, now known or hereafter invented, including photocopying and recording, or in any information storage or retrieval system, without permission, in writing from the **author/copyright** holder.

ISBN: 1-59971-429-9

Abstract

The purpose of this topic was to examine the controversy about male menopause. Many men do not believe that this is a major concern for their gender; however, various research articles have documented the validity of male menopause. Therefore, it is important for authors, healthcare providers, physicians, and the media to educate men about the realities of male menopause. Male menopause is also referred to as male climacteric, viropause, andropause, and andro deficiency. Male menopause and other associated words will be defined to assist the reader in better understanding the technical terminology that is associated with this disorder. This book examined how society, healthcare workers, and the media viewed male menopause, and it suggested, through research, why men have a hard time accepting that they too will experience menopause as they age. The goal of this book was to report the findings from this author's study in an effort to help others support men who are experiencing the signs and symptoms of male menopause. The method of obtaining the statistics for this study was the use of an independently designed questionnaire, with 19 questions, adapted from the research literature that focused on men between the ages of 20 to 75 years of age that lived in the Detroit-Metropolitan Area. There were 200 questionnaires distributed, with an expected response rate of 50%. The surveys were conducted from November 30, 2004 through January 8, 2005. An Excel spreadsheet was used to total the responses to each question. Each question had the same degree of weight. A statistical correlation was done by focusing on questions 1 through 6 to discern if men know or do not know about male menopause. Based on 100 percent, a percentage rating was assigned, and the results were identified in percentages for each question. After all of the statistics were analyzed, this

author either accepted or rejected the research question(s).

Acknowledgments

I want to thank my Lord and Savior, Jesus Christ for giving me the health, strength, courage, and wisdom to complete this book. I am grateful to have accomplished this goal. I wish to thank my husband, Clayton, and my children, Druervonn, TaKyesia, and Warner II for all of their encouragement, patience, and love. Your understanding and unwavering love has helped me get through some very tough times. Without your support and unselfish nature, I could not have completed this endeavor. To my beloved parents, John D and Daisy, my sister, Delores, and my grandson, LeRoyce, I love you and know that you all were with me in spirit, rest in peace. I am eternally grateful to you all.

Table of Contents

List of Figures

List of Tables

CHAPTER ONE

Introduction

It has been said that every person in the world is distanced from knowing everyone else by six degrees of separation. "Everyone on Earth is separated from anyone else by no more than six degrees of separation, or six friends of friends of friends" (Six Degrees of Separation, n.d., p. 1). This was before the advent of the internet, a tool that is spreading communicative accessibility to unimaginable ranges while still keeping people at an arm's length. People have replaced communicating with one another in person, with digital phones, monitors, and internet 'communities'. Families are spending less time at the dinner table and more time with electronic devices. Many important issues are not discussed with children, sex being only one issue. Today, society is multi-tasking and may be ignoring addressing important concerns with their children and spouses. Male menopause is one of those important discussions that generally do not occur. Men are not eager to broach this topic, on the other hand; women have less inhibition about discussing sex and other health issues.

Historically, women talk about their health problems with other. "Midlife women may seek health care to resolve . . . problems" (Kessenrich, 2000, p. 1). On the other hand, men have been programmed by societal norms to keep certain issues to themselves, especially those concerns society has deemed non-masculine. Schieszer (2004) states, "the issue [male menopause] is now becoming more mainstream in part because . . . so many men are finally beginning to discuss their experiences (p. 1). Men are expected to act a certain way, and to carry a certain role in the household and in the community. In most cases, this just leads to men carrying a heavier burden by keeping important concerns to themselves and dealing with it internally. Therefore, it is no surprise that men are less likely to talk about important health issues. Men are especially quiet about health concerns that deal with problems related to male sexuality, male breast cancer, and male menopause. "Times change and people change. . . . Men are now freer to discuss their sexual performance problems . . . without fear of being ridiculed or ignored" (Steidle, 2004, p. 3). Ironically, male avoidance of sex-related topics still exists, as demonstrated in the research literature and this study.

In years past, the physical implications of male menopause were unheard of. Part of the reason could stem from the fact that the term male menopause was not used. Instead, male menopause was identified by several other names, most likely unfamiliar to men. "This phenomenon has been variously termed 'male climacteric', 'andropause', 'viropause', and 'androgen decline in aging men" (Fatusi, A. O., Ljadunola, K. T., Ojofeitimi, E. O., et al., 2003, p. 1). Today, in order for men to be able to cope with male climacteric, men should endeavor to understand what this phenomenon means. It is hypothesized that 50% of men either deny or ignore the reality of male menopause. Menopause is widely known as a female condition, perhaps leaving men to believe that this condition does not occur in males. This study will shed light on the problem of many men being in denial about andropause or simply do not understand the dynamics connected with this condition.

Introduction of the Problem

A major concern is that many men do not accept or do not understand the concept of male menopause. Initiating the learning process means that men should understand the role their sexual organs play with their sexuality, aging, and menopause. Anatomically speaking, men's testicles are bilateral to the penis and are housed inside of the scrotum. "The penis is composed mainly of erectile tissue" (Thomas, 1997, p. 1433). Appendix A and B will provide visual diagrams of the anatomy of the male libido, which includes male sex-organs and testosterone production, a male sex hormone. Testosterone is produced in the interstitial cells of the testicles and by the adrenal cortex of the kidneys. Thomas (1997) states that the testis "is one of two reproductive glands located in the scrotum that produces the male reproductive cells (spermatozoa) and the male hormones testosterone" (p. 1927). Low testosterone levels can create a problem with men's libido. Low testosterone can also be an indicator of male menopause. Men should address their concerns with their physicians and seek advice that will offer them the best resolution for their problems.

The sex hormone, testosterone, is responsible for the stimulation of a man's libido. Testosterone "is essential for normal sexual behavior and the occurrence of erection" (Thomas, 1997, p. 1928). Once men gain the basic knowledge of their libido, and learn how their sexual organs function, they may begin to grasp the entire concept of male menopause prompting men to inquire about diagnosis and treatment.

A significant component of the treatment regimen could include hormone replacement therapy. Hormone replacement therapy (HRT) is a form of treatment that presents another area of controversy associated with menopause. As previously stated, understanding their anatomy will give men a better understanding of how HRT works. Treatment can enhance a healthier sex life and a happier intimate relationship.

Statement of the Problem

It is clear from the research literature that countless men are in denial about the reality of male climacteric. This is especially true of those living in lower-economic, urban environments/communities. Forrest (1993) asserts, "poverty indicates if adequate resources are available to educate men and provide them with the necessary resources to educate them about the aging process" (p.1). Chapter Two will assess if there is a correlation between ethnicity and/or income levels and men's understanding or awareness of male menopause.

This study will investigate if at least 50% of the participants are in denial about male menopause. Furthermore, this study will explore the percentage of males who are unaware of male menopause. Because of men's denial, men may make life decisions and choices that are driven by the life changes they are experiencing. Male menopause may be understood on a psychological level mainly because menopause is linked to end-of-life issues that men are not willing to address, especially those men 40 years of age or older. Men may begin to ponder issues like how long they will be sexually pleasing to their spouses, who will care for their spouses after they die, and how long they have left to live.

Background Information of the Study

Because of men's denial of male menopause, marriages, relationships, and families are being compromised. Moreover, men's failure to educate themselves puts them at a disadvantage for diagnosis, ways to address the signs and symptoms that they may be experiencing, and therapeutic options. New information has suggested that men's lack of knowledge about male menopause could be the cause of their disinterest in this disorder. Driedger (1998) states that "men just don't talk about it" (p.1).

Male menopause is a topic that most men are not willing to discuss openly, especially in the presence of other men. However, ignorance could be the major contributing factor why men do not know enough about andropause. "The first study on male andropause was published . . . in the mid-1940s, it's only recently that the U. S. medical community has taken notice of this condition" (Gearon, 2004, p. 1). Perchance some men think by not discussing its existence that it just might disappear. Driedger (1998) asserts, "it may be more effective for men to seek an expanded definition of manliness" (p.2). Driedger further suggest that manliness is measured not solely by societal norms. Manliness is also measured by how well men adjust to life changing events, such as a decline in sexual and physical abilities, intimacy in relationships, and aging. Men need to change their attitudes and begin rebuilding their personal relationships, which can take a lot of time and effort. More exposure and discussion about andropause can help bring men around to the possibility of accepting this condition.

Purposes of the Study

One of the purposes of this study is to determine the extent of male ignorance or denial of male menopause. The author will seek to discover the degree of understanding that men have about male menopause and for those that deny it and why. Further, the study will examine why this topic is not widely discussed in the medical community. "Andropause was described as a syndrome by a variety of medical experts as early as the 1940s. . . . And the discomfort men feel about discussing their symptoms have kept doctors from accepting the syndrome as a treatable condition" (Steidle, 2004, p.3). This study, through the research literature, will further suggest how proper diagnosis can allow men to choose a treatment modality that is appropriate to their needs. Many authors have written on this condition; however, three authors are quoted in much of the research pertaining to male menopause.

Conceptual Framework

The most noted authors and researchers, on this topic, are Diamond, J., Driedger, S. D., and Tan, R. S., who suggest that there is a link to male menopause and declining testosterone levels. Furthermore, the aforementioned authors support the belief that diagnosis and treatment is significant to alleviating symptoms and providing a healthier sex life. Additionally, Diamond, J., Driedger, S. D., and Tan, R. S., and other authors on this topic consistently evaluate effective ways to educate and encourage men to acknowledge that male climacteric exists within their gender. The afore-mentioned authors have done extensive research on male menopause, and they postulate one consistent factor. Men continue to ignore the implications of male climacteric even though there is sufficient literature that is available to them. Interestingly, men are more tolerant of the belief that only females experience menopause.

Research Questions

This study will answer the following research questions:

1. How many men are aware of the concept of male menopause?

2. How many men do not regard male menopause as reality?

3. How many men know at what age they are more likely to experience menopause?

4. Of those men who accept the reality of this condition, how many are willing to address the problems that male menopause may cause.

5. What causes men to deny male menopause?

Nature of the Study

Of the many medical issues that individuals have to address, one that has not been discussed at great length is male climacteric. The nature of this study is to identify from the existing literature what health risks, if any, are associated with male climacteric, the differences between female and male climacteric, and the signs and symptoms associated with male menopause. The method of obtaining the statistical data related to the research questions of this study will be the use of an independently designed questionnaire adapted from the research literature that focuses on men between the ages of 20 to 75 years of age that live in the Detroit-Metropolitan Area. The research design for this study is a preordinate, qualitative (pre & posttest), as well as cross-sectional descriptive study. The chosen population will vary in economic status, educational status, ethnicity, and careers. The questionnaire incorporated what this author read, in the research literature, and the issues and findings consistently quoted by the authors referenced. There were 200 questionnaires distributed, with an expected response rate of 50%. More information about the design and instrumentation of this study can be located in Chapter Three. This study will analyze why men have a hard time accepting that they too will experience menopause as they age.

Significance of the Study

The significance of this study will determine how much knowledge or ignorance of menopause exists among the men surveyed. Moreover, this study will help the healthcare community better communicate to men the reality of male menopause. This study will aid men's understanding that male menopause is a natural phase that occurs with aging, just like with female menopause. Men will gain a better understanding to why men's attitudes may be more of fear. Fear may disallow men from seeking an enhanced understanding about this condition. The major objective of this study is to educate as many men as possible about this inevitable life occurrence. The goal for this study is to report the findings of this study to help others support men who are experiencing the signs and symptoms of male menopause.

Definitions of Terms

The terminology and definitions used in this study will assist the reader in better understanding the technical terminology that is associated with this disorder. The terminology below defines andropause, libido, male climacteric, male menopause, midlife crisis, and testosterone:

1. Andropause is another term used to describe male menopause. Andro is defined by Thomas (1997) as a "combining form meaning man, male, or masculine" (p. 95). Moreover, andropause is more specifically related to males as it addresses the change of life that men will experience. Hollander and Samons (2003) define andropause "as a symptom complex in the presence of low testosterone levels" (p. 3).

2. Libido as defined by Thomas (1997) is "the sexual drive, conscious or unconscious" (p. 1103).

4. Male climacteric, as previously stated, is a transitional period in a man's life that usually occurs after the age of 40. Rose (2000) states that male menopause "is a more accurate descriptor of the man's gradual transformation during his forties and fifties" (p. 4). During this time, men experience a decline in their testosterone levels that usually go undetected mainly because many men are unaware of this phenomenon. Male climacteric "has been misunderstood by all. Both by physicians as well as patients themselves. Many physicians fail to recognize this syndrome, and often misdiagnose it for something else" (Tan, 2001, p. 27).

5. For so many years, male menopause was a term that had been misunderstood. This misunderstanding was mainly because menopause is closely associated with women and their cessation of menstruation and the inability to have children. "While menopause is relative *[sic]* easy to diagnose in women - - their menstrual period stops - - diagnosing male menopause, also known as andropause, in men is trickier" (Schieszer, 2004, p. 2). The aforementioned terms: male climacteric,

andropause, or male menopause has been used interchangeably based on their definitions being the same. Puskar (n.d.) states, "sometimes called *andropause*, male menopause is a decline in testosterone levels that can cause a loss of libido" (p. 118).

6. Midlife crisis according to Rose (2000) "tends to be an emotional or psychological shift" (p. 4).

7. Testosterone is defined as "an androgen isolated from testes of a number of animals including man and considered to be the principal testicular hormone produced in man. . . . It stimulates and promotes . . . normal sexual behaviors and the occurrence of erections" (Thomas, 1997, p. 1928).

Assumptions and Limitations

This study made the following assumptions:

1. Most men are in denial about male menopause.

2. Most men lack enough information to persuade them of the realities of male menopause.

3. Male physicians are apprehensive about discussing male menopause with their male clients.

4. The media and healthcare providers need to spend more efforts in educating men about menopause.

This study has determined the following limitations:

1. A quantitative approach is needed to validate the findings.

2. The population was limited to a specific geographical area.

3. Because of the sensitive nature of this topic, the participants may not answer the questions truthfully.

4. More time allotted to data collection can provide increase response numbers that will offer more insight to why men deny or disbelieve the existence of male menopause.

Organization of the Remainder of the Study

The remaining chapters provide information about male menopause, the methodology used in this study, data collection and results, and a summary of the study and its findings. Chapter Two will discuss the literature related to male menopause as well as methodologies used in studies similar to this one. Chapter Three describes the methodology used for this study. Chapter Four presents and analyzes the data collected. Chapter Five will offer conclusions from the data collected, report on the significance of the findings from this study, including the conclusions drawn in Chapter Four. Furthermore, Chapter Five will offer recommendations for future studies.

CHAPTER TWO

Literature Review

Male menopause is a transition from one phase of life into another. Therefore, it is significantly important and needs addressing. A review of the literature will give collaborating support that men actually transition to andropause as they age. Schieszer (2004) states, "I know men are interested in it and I know more men are showing up for diagnosis and treatment. . . . There is steady growth" (p. 4). It is worth noting that change is inherent in the human life cycle. From birth to death, an individual will experience many physical and psychological changes that may affect their health. Therefore, this study will acknowledge that a "healthier lifestyles may enable an increasing number of today's young and middle-aged adults to maintain a high level of physical functioning well into old age" (Papalia, Olds, & Feldman, 2001, p. 654).

Because male climacteric is as much of a reality for men as it is for women, men will also experience the same or similar life changes associated with this condition. In lay-terms, menopause is also called *the change of life*. Therefore, male menopause will be explored to educate men about *the change of life* as well as exploring how these changes occur. This study defines the terminology associated with male menopause, in Chapter One; this study also describes how the decline in male sex hormone production of testosterone is significant in the diagnosis of male climacteric; and more specifically; this study describes how testosterone affects the male libido. Furthermore, this study will propose and analyze the important life changing issues facing men, distinguish the differences between male and female climacteric, and finally, defend the reality that men as well as women experience menopause.

Although men are more aware of female climacteric, they may not be cognizant of male climacteric. This study will emphasize men's need to be educated about male climacteric. A review of the literature will validate the existence of male climacteric. Additionally, this study will analyze why men are in denial about the reality of male climacteric. This study will discuss what the research literature reports on men's understanding of menopause.

A well-informed public can be instrumental in helping men and women understand the changes that occur throughout the lifecycle. This study will address the importance of health care professionals and the media working together to educate men, who are the targeted population, about the probability of men experiencing andropause. Postgraduate Medicine (2004) indicates that "primary care physicians are probably in the best position to evaluate the andropause syndrome in aging patients" (p. 4). In addition to physicians educating men about menopause, Hollander & Samons (2003) bring to light the confusion about male menopause that can create more doubt in men's minds mainly because "recent controversy has erupted in the popular media over whether andropause is a normal state of aging that is being medicalized in attempt to sell pharmaceutical products" (p. 3). Viagra, Cialis, and Levitra are only a few sex-stimulating drugs being popularized in the media.

Taking sex-stimulating medication may allay men's fears about this transition in life. Menopause is believed to cause men's inability to sustain an erection, to cause men to feel sexually unpleasing to their mates, and to decrease men's desire for sex. Research has also shown that "men suffering from this 'syndrome' are said to experience increasing irritability, fatigue, and sluggishness, as well as a reduced interest in sex" (Wittmeier, 1999, p. 1). The aforementioned drugs can promote men's belief that they do not have problems with their libido or experiencing warning signs of male menopause. The quandary that men must face is if male menopause is real or not. Because of the debate on whether men experience menopause, research have been able to prove, through various documented theories, that this is a condition worthy of men's attention. If men accept and realize that menopause is a normal part of the aging process, they should initiate steps to learn more about male menopause.

The Aging Process and Menopause

Initially, menopause described the period when a woman's reproductive phase had ended; however, menopause is now associated with men. "Menopause, more often than not, is associated with women who experience a cessation of their menstrual cycle. However, the term is now being used to delineate the changes men experiences as they age" (Isaac, 2002, p. 1). It is of vital importance that men become educated to what male climacteric is and the implications it has on the aging process. It is important to mention that men "indicated it was a subject they did not think about, consciously at least" (LeShan, 1973, p. 76). Male climacteric is a condition that should be taken seriously because there are many internal and external changes that occur as men age.

There are physiological as well as psychological changes during male menopause that men fail to realize as being important. The physical aspects of aging alone can create turmoil for individuals transitioning through life. These physical changes include the

gradual loss of hair or thinning hair, the inability to obtain or sustain an erection, bone

decalcification, and various other health problems, some were previously mentioned.

Men should question if the causes are hormonal only, or are they related to other

problems. "Few would fault the thesis that the body does not work well when hormonal

substances are depleted" (Swanton, 1998, P. 1). These adverse effects can have serious

implications and, are in many instances, precursors to other health problems that need to

be addressed and treated.

LeShan (1973) states:

> The body does begin to 'depreciate', and we are stuck with that reality. But in the
>
> very process of accepting this fact and trying to do intelligent and creative things
>
> about it, we can open ourselves up to all kinds of new experiences that may be
>
> even more rewarding (p. 261).

Men not only have to cope with aging, they also have to cope with the *change of life,* in

addition to the obvious physiological, psychological, and psychosocial changes.

The *change of life* can be a time of enormous uncertainty. "Most middle-aged

men really believe, deep-down, that enthusiasm for hunting, fishing, boxing, and football

still take the measure of a *real* man [italics added]" (LeShan, 1973, p. 77). Unfortunately,

many men try to conceal the fact that they are going through a transformation by

becoming overly concerned with their physical attributes causing them to work hard at

trying to ensure that they appear masculine. For some men, the mirror can be considered

their foe because the mirror reflects reality. According to LeShan (1973) during an interview with a gentleman, he stated, "One day, while shaving, I saw myself in a sudden sharp flash of unrecognition – you know, like the man in the mirror was a total stranger I'd never seen before" (p. 79).

While interviewing another man, LeShan (1973) states:

When I used to pass a pretty young woman on the street, there was a sort of electricity between us -- a message that I found her very attractive, and that the feeling might be reciprocated. Lately I've noticed that this happens less and less often (p. 79).

The reality of aging, alone, can be difficult to deal with. LeShan (1973) asserts, "men did not want to think about middle age . . . . The large majority did not want to talk about it" (p. 76). LeShan (1973) further asserts, "high on the list of concerns and special sensitivities was the matter of remaining sexually attractive to women" (p. 79). Many men become preoccupied with their physical appearance. Therefore, men appear to look more at their outer shell than their overall health. The loss of muscle and the visible increase in weight could be an indicator for men to seek medical advice and to inquire about their testosterone levels. A quiz developed by Andropause.com prompts men to answer questions that can later be used to discuss testosterone and menopause with their healthcare practitioners. Refer to Appendix D.

Physiologically men may notice a decrease in muscle mass and an increase in body-fatness. "Testosterone . . . can boost muscle mass" (Lacayo & McLaughlin, 2000; p. 3). The additional fat is more noticeable around the waistline and is linked to decreasing testosterone levels in the blood. Mirkin (2002) asserts, "as men age from 50 to 70, their testosterone levels drop more than 40%, causing them to become fatter, and less sexual, muscular and assertive and have smaller, weaker bones" (p. 1). Moreover, Ahlborg (2003) asserts, "menopause was determined according to the definition established by the World Health Organization [as the period when] . . . age dependent reduction in bone mineral density accelerated after menopause with the highest bone loss found during the first 5 years following menopause" (p. 1). These findings are mainly due to the decreasing amounts of blood testosterone in men. Besides the decrease physical appearance, men are at risk for a decline in their cognitive capability.

Not only do men become heavier and less physically attractive, but also menopause can bring on a decrease in a person's mental abilities. A huge segment of the male population experiences gradual erosion in their mental capabilities. Of all the changes that men go through, mental lapses, senility, and other mental disorders are perhaps just as distressing as their decrease in libido. Smolensky & Lamberg (2000) state that "declining hormones also affect memory and cognition" (p. 136). Men should be made aware that menopause could be a lengthy process. It can begin many years before the overt signs and symptoms are noticed and can become progressively worse as a person ages. This will most likely cause men to notice they no longer have the ability to sustain an erection.

The most significant matter related to male menopause, besides the physical concerns associated with aging, is that most men fear erectile dysfunction. Erectile dysfunction or ED is considered a man's inability to obtain or maintain an erection. Not being able to perform adequately in bed can cause deep internal turmoil and sometimes it can result in the disintegration of one's marriage.

Rose (2000) affirms:

> Men have not been encouraged to sit with their feelings or to turn to others for help. The fear of inadequacy and emasculation drive him to keep his fears and emotions locked in, and he begins to push others away so that they don't see through his ruse. Marriages break up as spouses drift further and further apart, perhaps taking other partners in an attempt to find the support and openness they don't have with each other (p.195).

Therefore, it is understood that men need to understand the entire aging process and its affects. Research has indicated that men are slowly beginning to come to terms with the issue of male menopause, which could mean they are familiarizing themselves with the risks, signs and symptoms, and treatment for this disorder. Male menopause, left untreated, could be a precursor to a man having difficulty obtaining or sustaining an erection that can eventually lead to impotency. Therefore, it is important for men to know that "approximately 40% of men in their 40s, 50s and 60s will experience some degree of difficulty in attaining and sustaining erections, lethargy, depression, increased irritability, and mood swings that characterize male menopause" (Diamond, 2003, p. 1). Understanding fosters acceptance and can alleviate many fears. Erectile dysfunction is another component of why men may not broach the topic of male menopause.

Initially, ED was thought to be synonymous with impotency; however, literature indicates that ED is quite different. Smolensky & Lamberg (2000) state that erectile dysfunction was "once wrongly termed *impotence* [italic added]" (p.140). ED is known to affect men as they get older and as troubling as this fact may be, a man's sexual ability remains an important factor in defining his manliness. Foresta, Caretta, Garolla, & Rossato (2003) confirm, "erectile function progressively declines with age" (p.1). Communication is paramount because many misconceptions can hinder men from asking the appropriate questions and obtaining answers about the symptoms they may be experiencing.

In addition, men's fears may stem from a communication barrier between them and their physicians. Physicians should be able to talk with their clients in a way that will enhance their understanding about male menopause. Male menopause could be dealt with in a more efficient way if men were to take the responsibility for educating themselves about their bodies. Certainly, men are not expected to do this without the help of qualified individuals. Doctors and other health professionals should contribute their knowledge by giving men the information and support they need. Doctors and other health care professionals can assist men in understanding male menopause by educating them to their own libido and sexual anatomy. Men may not understand how their sexual organs function; and men may not know the role their anatomy plays with sexuality and menopause.

The impetus for men to understand male menopause is by first getting them to understand that there are various viewpoints and theoretical perspectives about this process. Male climacteric is a phenomenon not embraced by all men, health care professionals, or those who have written on this topic. The myriad theoretical perspectives on this health condition are clear evidence of the divergent views on male climacteric. Moreover, each author has his/her own vantage point on various issues associated with male climacteric or menopause. Various theoretical perspectives were discussed in Chapters One and Two. It will be apparent that some authors view male menopause, its associated symptoms, and the role of testosterone differently.

Male climacteric is a term used to describe the transitional period in a man's life that indicates a decrease in the male sex hormone testosterone. "The major effect of testosterone deficiency on sexuality seems to be loss of libido" (Rose, 2000, p. 102). . Testosterone is linked to a man's ability to procreate as well as his desire to have sexual intercourse. "Although fertility may not be dramatically affected, the hormonal changes that men go through from their thirties on are significant" (Rose, 2000, p. 3). To further the point, Spark (2000) affirms, "depression and testosterone insufficiency are two most common causes of decreased libido".

What might be frightening to men is that menopause usually signifies a decrease in sexual desire (libido) or sexual activity. As previously mentioned, men's fears can lead to stress, anxiety, and depression. Male menopause, in it self, could cause men to act in ways that mask their fears instead of choosing to educate themselves about this phenomenon. Tan (2001) annotates, "all changes bring about stress, and if stress is not managed well, it can be very disabling and even lead to depression" (p. 165). Providing treatment to alleviate depression or normalize blood testosterone levels may be all that is needed to restore sexual function in these men" (p. 111). Men should view menopause as a stage of life that is natural. Instead, many men may believe that menopause is a problem

that they need not address.

Men and Their Understanding of Andropause

Another reason why men may be apprehensive about accepting the concept of male climacteric is, for many years, the public has ignored the fact that men too experience menopause. Men's lack of knowledge could cause great harm to them later, even though "there is an increasing awareness of andropause and male sexual dysfunction among the general public and the health community. In contrast, very little attention is still being paid to male sexual issues" (Fatusi, Ijadunola, Adeyemi, et al., 2003, p. 3). Consequently, men not only have a hard time accepting male climacteric, they lack the understanding about the risks, signs and symptoms, and treatment for this disorder.

The adverse side effects of male climacteric, previously mentioned, could have far-reaching implications, if it is not diagnosed and treated. Cohen (2003) states, "it's a silent crisis among men *andropause [italics added]*" (p.1). As with male breast cancer, male menopause is a taboo topic. "A high proportion of men inadvertently deny the presence of these changes, especially sexually related ones, and suffer in silence" (Fatusi, Ijadunola, Adeyemi, et al., 2003, p. 26). Therefore, men act as if they are okay, while remaining silent. Women differ, because they will discuss almost anything with their doctors. Sometimes this means discussing their husbands concerns as well.

Therefore, the problem could be that men do not view or will not accept any of their life changes, as menopause. Ironically, research shows that men more readily accept that women experience menopause. There are certain issues, problems, or diseases that are considered female-dominated concerns, and historically women have owned these life-altering changes, such as breast cancer and menopause. Fatusi, Ijadunola, Adeyemi, et al. (2003) assert, "most women do not hesitate to complain about their mid-life crisis" (p. 2). For the most part, society, the media, and documented literature on male menopause are to some extent conflicting. The confusion and inconsistencies have given men a reason to disbelieve that there is any connection between men and menopause.

Recent reports have suggested that men's lack of knowledge about male menopause could indicate their uncertainty about this disorder. Driedger (1998) states that "the American writer admits that male menopause is a misnomer, although it is convenient shorthand for the male middle-life slump" (p.1). Men's lack of awareness regarding male menopause might be contributed to the conflicting data on this topic. Some researchers have made the argument that men do not experience menopause and this allows men to believe that their apprehensions about male menopause are valid. At the same time, other authors have shown, through research, that menopause does occur in men.

Research literature indicates that men may lack the understanding of andropause and sometimes are not able to recognize it, or worst, deny its existence. The denial may be, in part, due to the conflicting research data or related to medical professionals not being familiar with this disorder. "The current paradigm in medicine is that there is no biological basis for behavioral changes in midlife men so it is ignored" (Andropause, n.d., p.2). Therefore, the question is worth asking and answering, how should men assert themselves to learn about a problem that they may not believe exist? "Men need to realize and accept that this disorder exists" (Andropause, n.d., p. 2). Once men have a better quasi understanding of this disorder then they can begin learning more about the signs and symptoms associated with andropause and the available treatment. Another factor than can create confusion for males accepting menopause is that some signs and symptoms are similar to depression in men. "The second form of this syndrome (male menopause) is more insidious since it occurs gradually. It is often confused with male midlife psychological adjustment disorders because it exactly mimics depression in midlife men" (Andropause, n.d., p. 2). Chapter One introduced some signs and symptoms of depression and how depression is linked to male menopause. This chapter will expound on the specific signs and symptoms of male menopause.

Do Men Ignore the Signs and Symptoms of Male Menopause?

Men are not entirely to blame for the non-acceptance of male menopause. In part, society has to shoulder some of the responsibility due to the social stigma attached to this disorder. "Underneath the whole 'male menopause syndrome' may be a man who feels he is losing control" (Driedger, 1998, p. 2). If men ignore any signs and symptoms associated with menopause, they will increase the delay in treatment. Schieszer (2004) estimated that five percent of four million to five million American men diagnosed with low testosterone are treated in order to protect against the chance of decreased libido or impotency.

Research has indicated that both men and women have gender-specific hormones that decrease as they age. In women, the hormone estrogen is evaluated to determine if they are either perimenopausal or menopausal. "The chief sexual hormones in women are estrogen" (Smokensky and Lambert, 2000, p. 124). In men, their testosterone levels are evaluated to establish their likelihood of being perimenopausal or menopausal.

Smokensky and Lambert (2000) affirm, "the chief one (hormone) is testosterone, made mainly by the testes" (p. 124). Obtaining hormone levels are simple and painless. The testing procedure for checking estrogen and testosterone is a standard blood test that is obtained by drawing serum levels of the aforementioned hormones. "The diagnosis is quite simple - - namely measuring . . . free testosterone blood levels" (Andropause, n.d., p. 2). Testing a man's (testosterone) or a woman's (estrogen) hormone level can determine if he/she is perimenopausal or menopausal. This screening process could be important to both men and women in the attempt of maintaining a healthy sex life.

According to Schieszer (2004), "currently, a small number of studies have shown that testosterone replacement in men who have low levels of the hormone can improve libido and enhance sexual function" (p.3). If men were more cognizant of the particular problems and sought early detection, many of the stereotypes, misconceptions, and physiological problems could be dealt with more productively. However, as long as the ego continues to foster doubt about the very existence of male menopause, men will continue to deny the psychological as well as physiological problems associated with this disorder.

A plethora of theories and research has been analyzed in an attempt to explain why men are in denial about andropause. "First men need to disassociate their ego from their testicles. Men needs *[sic]* to realize and accept that this disorder exists . . . , and that it can be treated" (Andropause, n.d. p. 2). Once men begin to face this concept, then they will be better prepared to deal with andropause.

What Must Men Face When Dealing With Andropause?

Men facing andropause should first confront their egos and admit that male climacteric is a natural biological change that occurs with aging. Perry (2001) affirms, "among men, some sexual problems may increase with age" (p. 143). Moreover, "the male ego doesn't usually ever want to admit to having a problem" (Schieszer, 2004, p. 1). Men want to maintain a macho image that has been perpetuated for years as a sign of masculinity. Schieszer (2004) asserts, "men want to be macho" (p. 1). If men allow themselves to accept that male menopause exist, men are then faced with addressing sexual concerns, i.e. decreasing libidos or sex-drive, difficulty with erections, and not being capable of sexually satisfy their partners. "Having a suitable partner is a major factor in whether and how often older people engage in sexual activity" (Perry, 2001, p. 145). Sex does not have to end because of menopause. Men may have to learn more about sexually stimulating ways to continue enjoying sex and pleasing their mates. "Normal sexual function is much more than being able to have penile erection or an ejaculation. There is also the dimension of libido, the feeling of desire, drive and energy associated with sexual stimulus" (Tan, 2001, p. 102). Therefore, a major hindrance to why men may ignore indications of menopause may be attributed to their egos. Because of their avoidance, men may not learn effectively how to deal with the reality that menopause will eventually occur.

Moreover, when ego borders on de-validating the man's masculinity and sexuality, the ego will win out causing men to deny that male menopause exists. "The male ego doesn't usually ever want to admit to having a problem. Men want to be macho and if they have a problem, they just don't want to talk about it. . . . But the guys will only talk to me [the doctor] in private" (Schieszer, 2004, p. 1).

Does the Male Ego Play an Integral Role in Men's Denial of Andropause?

Being in a constant state of denial about male menopause could result in men looking for their lost youth or attempting to hang on to it. Men could resort to acting irresponsibly. Men have been know to date younger women, divorce their wives, wear their hair in ponytails, pierce their ears, and do all manner of things, which negate the reality of the aging process or their own mortality. LeShan (1973) asserts, "for the first time I can really understand why men my age leave their wives for younger women. It's to reassure themselves and tell the world they've still got 'it' – whatever *it is* [italics added]" (p. 79). *It* is sometimes called midlife crisis.

Midlife crisis has been described as men "acting out" or attempting to "recapture" their youth. In addition to the aforementioned changes, "they're buying sports cars, growing ponytails, and leaving their wives to take up with younger women" (Rose, 2000, p. 4). This phase of "acting out" is an attempt to avoid the horrible reality of aging. Rose (2000) states, "some men 'act out' and have a last go at turning back the clock. [Most men do not know that this is] the midlife crisis [that] tends to occur earlier than andropause" (p.4). Men's "acting out" may be a way for men's egos to allow them to deny the changes that are taking place in their bodies.

Ego is one assertion why men deny that andropause exists. Being overly preoccupied with oneself is defined as egocentric, a characteristic socially attributed to males. Goodwin (2001) explains, "from a distance it will sound like a substantial whine, produced by million of male narcissists complaining: *it's not fair, I want it all* [italics added]" (p.2). Consequently, the egocentric aspect is that men believe menopause is a female-specific disorder. To accept that male menopause is a reality *means* that men also have to recognize that they would inevitably experience the signs and symptoms associated with male menopause.

The concept of male menopause can be intimidating in its own right. Hence, it is understandable that a decrease in libido, erectile dysfunction, a lack of sexual motivation, and the potential inability to satisfy their mates sexually can only heighten men's fears. A male afflicted with male menopause is considered the antithesis of the male ego. Chase (1998) asserts, "many middle-aged men seek supplements to boost energy and sexual zest" (p.2). "Because they are supposed to be strong, men deny they have a problem with their sexuality and don't understand the relationship with depression" (Diamond, 2003, p. 1).

Interestingly, male menopause has not been easy to diagnose in all men because it can resemble depression. "The most common problem associated with male menopause is depression which is closely related to impotence and problems with male sexuality" (Diamond, 2003, p. 1). An important factor of male climacteric is depression that could be related to men having to face their pending loss of libido or manhood. In addition, male climacteric signifies the transition from young man to mature man. At this transitional phase, death and dying issues also may become a reality.

Diamond (2003) delineates:

1. 80% of all suicides in the US are men

2. The male suicide rate at midlife is three times higher as compared to women; and for men over age 65 suicides is seven times higher.

3. The history of depression makes the risk of suicide seventy-eight times greater

4. 20 million Americans will experience depression sometimes in their lifetime

5. 60-80% of depressed adults never get professional help, and

6. It can take up to ten years and three health professionals for a proper diagnose of male menopause

Diamond (2003) asserts, "men are more likely to act out their inner turmoil while women are more likely to turn their feelings inward" (p. 2). The aforementioned author delineates the following signs of male menopause that is also linked to depression:

1. Blaming others

2. Irritable and angry

3. Inflated ego

4. Initiates conflict

5. Covertly or overtly hostile

6. Feels suspicious and cautious

7. Attacks others when feeling hurt

8. Restless and easily agitated

9. Feels the world is setting them up to fail

10. Experiences insomnia

11. Frustrated, if not praised enough

12. Frightened to converse about weaknesses and doubts

13. Compulsive timekeeper

14. Strong fear of failure

15. Need to be "top dog" and to feel safe

16. Chooses alcohol, television, sports, and sex to self-medicate

17. Believe their problems could be solved only if their (spouse, co-worker,

parent, and/or friend) would treat them better

18. Constantly, wonder "am I being loved enough"?

Diagnosis for male menopause should start prior to any manifestations of

psychological symptoms, such as moodiness, depression, irritability, and/or a decreased

libido. This may be achieved by men being educated enough to address their symptoms

with their physicians early. Once men initiate dialogue with their doctors about the

symptoms that they are experiencing, physicians should start monitoring their male

clients' testosterone levels on a regular basis. Andropause (n.d.) states, "perhaps, more

important, physicians, psychologists, and other health providers need to be taught about

this condition" (p.2) and pass the information on to their male clients. Men being aware

of the signs and symptoms could prompt them to seek interventions at the first indication.

"It is important not to dismiss . . . changes related to the andropause" (Tan, 2001, p. 12).

Any of the aforementioned signs and symptoms, including those indicating the

possibility of depression, should prompt a man to seek professional help to have the

possibility of menopause ruled-out. Spark (2000) indicates that treatment can be initiated

if men voice their concerns about growing old. Men need to be more proactive with

discussing their concerns with their practitioners, especially when they experience any symptoms that are different or abnormal. Schieszer (2004) affirms, "the man has to have a relationship with his physician and his physician has to be an educator and have a thorough discussion of what are the man's symptoms" (p. 3). Diagnosis is considered the first step in alerting men about menopause; however, it does not prevent this disorder.

Treatment is needed to ward off symptoms that men may be having. Treatment is usually delayed because many men have not accepted the reality that they can be diagnosed with menopause. Eastman (2004) states, "men are the biggest deniers and the last to go to doctors" (p. 16). Denial of male menopause delays treatment that can decrease and/or eliminate unnecessary symptoms. "Currently, a small number of studies have shown that testosterone replacement in men who have low levels of the hormone can improve libido and enhance sexual function" (Schieszer, 2004, p.3). Hence, if men are treated early, they could enhance the quality of their sex lives and possibly eliminate many, if not all, of the symptoms associated with male menopause. Perhaps the most difficult part of the treatment process is getting men to come to grips with the fact that male menopause will occur whether they accept it or not. "Deep inside every man is the desire to remain young" (Tan 2001, p. 17). The need to stay youthful could give men an excuse to ignore symptoms that would inevitably delay diagnosis and treatment. Treatment could be extremely beneficial by restoring men with a healthier libido. Men need to inquire about their treatment choices. Men's denial or lack of understanding for this phenomenon can put them at risk for missing very important indicators.

Do Men Lack the Understanding of Male Menopause?

As previously stated, men doubt that they have a chance of experiencing male climacteric; therefore, men may not find it necessary to consult a physician to have a baseline blood analysis. Eastman (2004) states, "men are the biggest deniers and the last to go to doctors" (p. 16). It is vitally important that men, who are in the age range for male menopause, 40 years old and older, receive the proper diagnosis, by a qualified physician, as this is the first line of defense in treating this condition. Eastman (2004) states that it is dangerous "when men do not get check-ups and needed treatment" (p. 16). By being proactive and having their hormone levels checked, men could alleviate their fear of impotency and receive assistance in planning a medical regimen that can enhance sexual activity. Hollander & Samons (2003) assert that more needs to be known about "which men should be tested for low testosterone and which are candidates for replacement therapy" (p.5).

Menopause has the stigma of being non-masculine; therefore, men do not want to broach the subject of male menopause. Fatusi, Ijadunola, Adeyemi, et al. (2003) state, "male menopause . . . has a negative impact on the quality of life in men" (p. 2). Most researchers concur that many men tend to underestimate male menopause by focusing entirely on becoming older and a decrease in physical activity. Wittmeier (1999) found that "recent publicity about the existence of a male form of menopause has added to men's anxiety over aging (p. 1). Revisiting the statement that men may not understand or are not willing to accept the concept of male menopause indicates that additional education is needed. "Many men . . . dismiss the symptoms of menopause as *women stuff* [italics added]" (Driedger, 1998, p.1). It would be advantageous if men had access to information that would assist them in learning how the biological changes could affect them physiologically and psychologically, as they age. There is a greater potential for harm if men continue to allow their egos to hinder them from learning as much as possible about andropause.

Some potential harms of male menopause is that men could experience depression, memory loss, and a decreased libido, which are all reasons to begin to encourage men to focus more seriously on male menopause and its treatment. Driedger (1998) states menopause "is a matter of 'mind over manliness' . . . . It may be much more tempting to just pop a pill" (p. 2). The pill of choice for this condition appears to be Viagra. Although, sex-stimulating medications may appear to alleviate the symptoms and increases libido, men should know that there is no cure for this disorder. Viagra and the other sex-stimulating drugs are only effective in treating the symptoms associated with decreased libido.

Aside from the male ego playing a role in men's dismissal of male menopause, there are psychosocial issues relating to ethnicity and/or income levels that could also present additional problems. Forrest (1993) indicates that there is a correlation between the availability of medical resources and income. Forrest looked at non-Hispanic whites, who were determined to have higher incomes. The non-Hispanics had more medical resources and information available to them as compared to those classified as low-income, black, and/or Hispanic. Men's lack of understanding about male menopause could be linked, in part, to ethnicity and those in a lower economic/income bracket.

These factors could hinder some men from getting the type of professional help they need, further compromising their ability to be properly educated about male menopause. Forrest (1993) asserts that poverty, economic status, race, and ethnicity indicates the importance of focusing on the delivery of service and education by directing efforts to providing women and men with needed information and services and to assess possible effects.

Females' vs. Males' Understanding of Male Menopause

As with female menopause, male menopause is considered a poignant change in a person's life. Stuttaford, Simson, & Zaleski (1997) state that both sexes need to "embrace their midlife passage and to move on to their *second adulthood* [italics added] as mature mentors" (p.2). During menopause, as with females, males will experience a decrease in libido (sex drive), mood swings, and a decreased interest in intimacy. Driedger (1998) writes, "both sexes . . . may experience mood swings, irritability, and waning sexual desire during the change of life" (p. 1). Because women are more receptive to hearing about menopause, women prepare for this period of change in their lives, while men deny or doubt they will ever experience menopause. "The process is more elusive in men . . . , kicking in later-usually in the 50s and 60s". (Driedger, 1998, p. 1). Research indicates that by the time men reach age 50, they have already begun the search for the proverbial fountain of youth.

Many females are aware that men also go through *the change of life,* as it is commonly known. Marc R. Rose, M.D. wrote a book in 2000 that addressed females' understanding of male menopause, titled, *A Women's Guide to Male Menopause.*

Nonetheless, "menopause, more often than not, is associated with women who experience a cessation of their menstrual cycle. However, the term is now being used to delineate the changes men experiences as they age" (Isaac, 2002, p. 1). Conversely, it has not been easy to convince men that they, too, experience *the change of life.*

"Male menopause, or andropause, is a complex clinical syndrome with several psychiatric manifestations, coexisting with low testosterone levels or hypoganadism. One area of controversy concerns whether andropause is a real clinical syndrome or a normal aspect of aging" (Hollander & Samons, 2003, p.2). Females readily seek professional advice whenever they experience physical and/or psychological changes. Research has shown that there is a vast difference in how the two genders go about seeking medical advice. Rose (2000) explains, "it's almost always the women in the family who seeks information on health and then applies it. And, fortunately, the man tends to listen when the woman of the family makes a health-care decision" (p. vii). Because women are more proactive in seeking medical information and passing the information on to men, more research is needed to determine how to involve men in participating in their healthcare.

First, those individuals that are well informed about male menopause need to educate men that menopause does not only affect women. Driedger (1998) states that the need "to guide men, and their mates, through the *unspeakable passage [italics added]*" (p.1). Hence, men are not singled out as the only gender to struggle with their egos concerning menopause. "There are many more similarities than differences between the male and female midlife passage" (Stuttaford & Simson, 1997, p. 1). This passage of life can be just as difficult for women.

If men were to disclose their symptoms, as openly as women, they would discover more about menopause. Despite the differences, menopause manifests itself similarly in both genders. Therefore, it is important to describe the similarities and differences because they demonstrate that not only women experience menopause, but also how it manifest itself in men.

The Similarities and Differences of Female and Male Menopause

The literature reports that there are more correlations to female and male menopause than men are aware. "There are many more similarities than differences between the male and female midlife passage" (Stuttaford, G., Simson, M., & Zaleski, J., 1997, p. 1). However, the most noticeable differences for those women going through menopause are they may notice a decline than a cessation of their menstrual cycles. Once women's menstrual cycles cease, they no longer can become pregnant. Conversely, in the case of men, they gradually experience a decline in their hormone levels much later than women. Eventually, men who have low testosterone levels will notice a decrease in their libido. Men's low testosterone will eventually render them unable to impregnate women, as they age. Stuttaford, G., Simson, M., and Zaleski, J. (1997) assert, "the two significant differences are that men can continue to procreate, and that women's hormonal changes are much more rapid and acute than men's" (p. 1). The similarities, for both genders, are noted in men and women's reported signs and symptoms. When men discuss what they experience, it usually is the same or similar to what women report. Driedger (1998) explains, "both sexes . . . may experience mood swings, irritability and waning sexual desire during the change of life. The process is more elusive in men, kicking in later" (p.

1). Studies have shown that the transition or change of life is more gradual in men than in women. Therefore, understanding this transition can be vital to men's health and sexual vitality. Men's understanding of the psychosocial implications of male menopause can significantly help them as they transition through this phase of life.

The Psychological Implications Affecting Menopausal Men

The psychological aspect of male menopause can be extremely stressful and depressing for men. "Testosterone treatment might improve depressed mood [sic] in older men who have low levels of bioavailable testosterone" (Barrett-Connor, Von Muhlen, & Kritz-Silverstein, 1999, p.1). Researchers have shown that men do not want to admit something is wrong with their sex lives. Conceivably, Mayer (1978) indicates that if men were aware that the statistics prove that males attain their sexual peak at eighteen, then their sexual peak declines steadily thereafter. Perhaps, if men understood that their sexual peak will begin to decline at an early age as well as knowing this is a natural process of life, this could alleviate some of their apprehension. With this knowledge, men may better deal with these facts instead of trying to avoid addressing midlife issues, such as menopause. As such, men would understand why they experience a waning desire for sex and/or that they do not engage in sexual intercourse as they did when they were younger. "Loss of sexual vigor is a common problem for men as they age. . . . More often, a sexual slowing down can be attributed to a combination of physical problems that occur as a natural consequence of aging" (Spark, 2000, p. 369). One way men can compensate for their decrease in sexual prowess is to learn new ways of pleasing their mates during intercourse. McCarthy and McCarthy (1998) state, "only one of six

American men has received an adequate sex education" (p. 2). From an early age,

individuals learn that sex is a natural act that can be an enormous source of enjoyment.

Perhaps, knowing this is what causes men awful fears over facing menopause and

admitting to their deficiencies in the bedroom.

Interestingly, men usually do not hesitate acknowledging that women experience

menopause, while at the same time denying experiencing menopause themselves. "Men

who have watched this whole process, or who are in the middle of helping a loved one

through it, may have breathed a sigh of relief that they don't have to go through it

themselves" (Rose, 2000, p.3). A male that Gould, Petty, and Jacobs (2000) interviewed

about male menopause stated, "I really do not find the analogy of the female menopause

helpful in understanding or trying to manage the problems of senescence in men"

Coming to terms with the realism of aging can be very traumatic for men.

Accepting this reality can create additional psychological problems, such as denial, anger,

infidelity, and bazaar behaviors. Hodges (2003) states, "the ageing male is generally

presented as a kindly, if feeble, old grandfather" (p.1). Hodges depiction of the middle-

aged man is quit different from what other researchers have documented in the

aforementioned texts. LeShan (1973) asserts, "men are far more unhappy about middle

age . . . and are much less in touch with these feelings" (p. 76). Menopause is known to

begin as early as 40 or 50. Many men may not consider themselves as old, middle-aged,

or a candidate for menopause. The denial could stem from the fact that men between the

ages of 40 to 50 are not willing to concede to the aging process. "In reality, there may

come a point when we have to accept things just as they are. After all, we are but mortals, and the Andropause is only one of the many chapters in our lives" (Tan, 2001, p.175).

Men are more likely to ignore this phenomenon and find ways to challenge this theory by

attempting to remain youthful and energetic. An impetus for men wanting to believe they

are still young and active could be their way of avoiding end of life concerns linked to the

aging process.

End of Life Issues Influencing Men Dealing with Menopause

In addition to all of the concerns that have been stated beforehand, such as,

irritability, mood swings, waning sexual desires, increased weight, and other age-specific

issues, men also have to confront end of life issues. LeShan (1973) asserts, "another man

told me that he felt middle-aged *when I knew the only place I was 'going' was toward the*

cemetery [italics added]" (p. 79). Clearly, many men find it difficult to accept the realism

of menopause or they deny it altogether. Menopause compounded with end-of-life issues

can cause men to experience severe mood swings. From all of the problems that men may

experience during their transitional phase, mood swings can cause many conflicts, which

can be devastating to their relationships. This conflict stems mainly from man's

apprehensions and refusal to be screened for menopause. "The underlying problems must

be found through diagnostic procedures before treatment can be suggested. A physical

examination always includes a medical and sexual history" (Perry, 2001, p.151). Mood

swings can be an unconscious way to deal with menopause on top of dealing with the

end-of-life issues man must be facing in silence.

Perry (2001) asserts:

> Over the course of a lifetime, men face a variety of inevitable stresses that create
> emotional responses. Dealing with death and dying presents some of life's greatest
> emotional stress.... *Bottled up* [italics added] emotions can lead to depression,
> withdrawal from friends and society, sudden irrational outbursts, feelings of anger
> and resentment . . . and even physical illness (p. 132).

Most men will never admit that they experience mood swings. Rose (2000) states,
"men don't have . . . hormonal cycles, and can go for years and years without dealing
with difficult emotional issues" (p. 9). Men's emotional state may stem from the
overwhelming ideation that they should consider andropause, while at the same time
address issues about their mortality.

The Media and Male Menopause

More recently, there have been news telecasts, coverage in newspaper articles,
journals, and books that have discussed specific issues pertaining to andropause: such as,
signs and symptoms, diagnosis, and treatment. "With publicity and media attention,
momentum is building" (Newman, 1996, p. 1). There is more media coverage currently
as compared to yesteryear. "The concept of 'male menopause' is being popularized"
(Newman, 1996, p. 1). Male menopause is becoming less and less of a taboo topic. "The
issue is now becoming more mainstream in part because . . . so many . . . men are finally
beginning to discuss their experiences" (Schieszer, 2004, p.1). Unfortunately, men are
still not buying in as much as they should, which could cause health problems later in
life. Schieszer (2004) states, "I think it is still in the closet but, it is gradually coming out

of the closet" (p. 2). As stated earlier, the role of the media is very important in dispersing information to men about male menopause. Through television broadcasts, newspapers, and journals, the subject of male menopause and the importance of men taking an active role in learning about important health issues have increased their awareness about this disorder.

What is the Role and Responsibility of the Media?

The media has a greater responsibility for disseminating the information because of its ability to reach a large population. Reputable individuals, such as doctors, nurses, and other health care practitioners must ensure that the media receives adequate and credible information. Axley (2003) indicates the need to move toward menopause symptom management by promoting a multi-disciplinary approach. It then becomes the responsibility of men to utilize the information better to educate themselves on the subject of andropause. A better understanding of male menopause will help men seek additional information concerning prevention, screening, diagnosis, and treatment. There is a limit to the responsibilities of the media; i.e. reporting the information to men about andropause. Men need to go a step further and take more responsibility for their health. Men can take additional responsibility by investigating all the possibilities related to their gender risks associated with menopause. Schieszer (2004) states, "I think this is where a man has to have a relationship with his physician and his physician has to be an educator and have a thorough discussion of what are the man's symptoms" (p.3). The media has been a perpetual influence in informing people about various health issues and now have turned the focus to informing men about andropause. "With publicity and media attention, momentum is building" (Newman, 1196, p. 1). Since andropause is becoming less of a prohibited topic, men are becoming more receptive to learning as much as possible about male menopause. Newfound cooperation from men allows nurses, doctors, and other health care personnel to take advantage of the opportunity to discuss male climacteric with men.

The Role of Nurses and Auxiliary Health Care Teams

It cannot be over emphasized that nurses along with other health care teams need to ensure that the media get reliable information circulated to men. With the aid of nurses and other qualified individuals addressing andropause, men will receive the necessary information to assist them in learning more about this disorder. "Nurses should be aware of the chronology and physiology of menopause" (Kessenrich, 2000, p. 1). A better-informed male population would be better poised to confront male menopause, thus making men better prepared to choose the best medical strategy and/or therapy that will properly address male menopause. Education will assist men in selecting the appropriate health care providers to begin the process of screening and prevention. Health professionals, including nurses, could play a significant role in bringing this vital issue to the forefront of male medical concerns. Nurses can do so by encouraging men to seek proper screening. "A screening test . . . can determine the risk for this disease (disorder)" (Kessenrich, 2000, p. 2). Nurses need to contribute educate men about the research addressing male menopause, then more men will be better informed about this disorder. "Nurses must understand the physiological changes of menopause and be aware of the important role they themselves can play in promoting the health of midlife" (Kessenrich, 2000, p. 1).

Undeniably, the topic of male menopause is complex and controversial. Therefore, it is no surprise why health professionals find it perplexing and are not fully aware of how menopause affects men. Schieszer (2004) cites the following case about an Illinois man, Dave O'Neal:

Was totally uninterested in sex and had very low energy levels. O'Neal went to several doctors and even a therapist but no one could tell him what was wrong. Eventually O'Neal was diagnosed with androgen deficiency, a problem of low testosterone levels in the body, also known as male menopause (p.1).

Research and Its Connection to Male Climacteric

Research supports the veracity of male climacteric. "Approximately 40% of men in their 40s, 50s, and 60s will experience some degree of difficulty in attaining and sustaining erections, lethargy, depression, increased irritability, and mood swings that characterize male menopause" (Diamond, 2003, p. 1). Not only has research validated this phenomenon, but it can also inform men about this life-changing event. Male menopause is not new, and there have been many studies about the need to educate men concerning this disorder. "The last few years have seen an increase in scientific interest in andropause, or menopause" (Hollander, 2003, p.1). Therefore, men have had the information available to them. However, many men have most likely, because of the social stigma, chosen not to educate themselves or talk with other men about this disorder. Stuttaford, Simson, and Zaleski (1997) suggested that mid-life men stop clinging to their youth and embrace the truth about male menopause, in order to educate younger men. Menopause is a natural biological event in a person's life that, when understood should, be embraced and not seen as a curse.

Hollander and Samons (2003) assert:

[Their] article addresses the complex clinical syndrome of male menopause, or andropause. Recent research on this topic has determined that this is a common and rarely treated condition, but has generated some controversy about whether or not this is just a normal part of aging (p. 5).

Through research, much has been learned about male menopause. Now, the task is convincing men to ask questions, review the research available to them, and discuss their option with their physicians.

How Convincing is the Research Associated to Male Menopause?

The reported research literature on male menopause is convincing because researchers have spelled out exactly what male menopause is and what men should watch for as they age. "Some researchers are taking seriously the still controversial notion of 'male menopause', a constellation of physical changes" (Richard & McLaughlin, 2000, p. 5). Moreover, "an astounding 57 million American men will experience menopause by the year 2020" (Lord, 2000, p.1). Hollander and Samons (2003) further confirm that "andropause remained an unstudied subject for years, but more recently; research in this topic has seen a marked increase" (p. 2). Men can learn more about this disorder by reading various research studies in order to convince them that menopause is not exclusive to females. Schieszer (2004) documented the comments of "Dr. Larry

Lipshultz, a professor of urology at Baylor College (who) says . . . men . . . will soon be

changing their minds once they are better educated" (p. 4). Research not only addresses

menopause, it also describes the effects of testosterone on men's sexual proficiency.

The Action and Importance of Testosterone

The action and importance of testosterone is mostly related to how a boy develops

into a man by causing male characteristics to develop, including his libido. "It's

testosterone that we understand and misunderstand as the essence of manhood" (Lacayo

& McLauglin, 2000, p. 2). Lacayo and McLaughlin (2000) further state, "It's the

hormone responsible for many things male, and levels peak between the ages of 15 and

30" (p. 9). Additionally, Lacayo and McLauglin (2000) delineate the actions of

testosterone: (a) stimulates the brains ability to concentrate, (b) increases men's libido or

sex drive, (c) stimulates hair growth on various parts of the body, (d) is responsible for

deepening men's voices, (e) aids in strengthening bone mass, (f) stimulates development

of male sex organs, (g) helps with men developing muscle mass, and (h) decreases the

number of fat cells in men. The goal is to have testosterone, produced by the endocrine

system, at a stable level in the body to defend against any possibilities of disharmony

with nature resulting in adverse psychological and/or physiological symptoms.

Rose (2000) states the following:

The hormonal, or endocrine, system is as finely tuned as the world's best

symphony orchestra. Each element is integrated into the whole, and each hormone

plays its role just as each musician plays his instrument. The endocrine system's job is to continually produce subtle adaptations in a man's body as the environment he lives in changes (p. 5).

Testosterone levels peak at a certain age and then testosterone levels begins to decline as a man ages. Unbeknownst to some, women have a small amount of testosterone in their bodies, but not as much as men. Men need to ask their doctors about their testosterone levels and learn of its actions.

Normal Testosterone Levels and Its Significance

Women's testosterone levels are much lower than men's; mainly that is why testosterone is classified as a male sex hormone. Normal testosterone levels for men, according to Lacayo and McLauglin (2000) are reported to be, on average, 260 to 1,000 nanograms per deciliter of blood or serum. Both, men and women are born with specific amounts of serum testosterone. Comparatively, for women, the levels are much lower, 15-70 nanograms per deciliter of blood. For both genders, the importance of normal levels of testosterone is homeostasis. "Both homeostasis and chronobiology are valid. Homeostasis mechanisms reveal the body's impressive facility for self-correction" (Smolensky & Lambert, 2000, p. 16). During menopause, homeostasis can be hard to obtain because of the changes that are occurring in the man's body. In some cases, exogenous hormones have to be substituted in order to bring balance back and decrease untoward symptoms. "Serum testosterone levels decline gradually and progressively with aging. . . . Testosterone supplementation may prevent or reverse the effects of aging" (Gruenewald & Matsumoto, 2003, p. 1). If men, as they age, continue to dismiss this phenomenon they will not notice that their testosterone levels have decreased. More importantly, they will not be aware of the psychological and physiological changes associated with male climacteric. "So they can produce a roller coaster of emotional and physical effects, from a burst of energy, snappishness, and libido in the first days to fatigue and depression later" (Lacayo & McLauglin, 2000, p. 2).

On the contrary, younger men are known to have a healthier sex life because of their higher testosterone levels; however, as men age, their desire for sex will eventually lessen. "The age-related decrease in anabolic hormone production coincides with loss of muscle mass . . . and diminished vigor, stamina, and sexual function" (Spark, 2000, p. 380). Therefore, it is important that those qualified to educate men about male climacteric should attempt to discuss the inevitable changes that young men will experience as early as possible. Early education about this disorder will encourage young men to monitor their blood testosterone levels and watch for signs and symptoms that may necessitate medical attention. With early diagnosis of andropause, men could receive appropriate interventions, while maintaining a healthy libido.

The Implications that Male Menopause have on Men's Libido

Researchers contend that as testosterone levels decrease, the probability of a healthy libido decreases as well. However, what men should be made aware of is that "there are also many reports of individuals who wrote on their improved libido following testosterone . . . treatments" (Tan, 2001, p. 42). Men could unconsciously ignore their decline in sexual pleasures in lieu of facing the reality that they may be entering menopause. Dismissal of this phenomenon is especially true if men do not believe that

menopause could happen to them. Driedger (1998) asserts, "it may be more effective for men to seek an expanded definition of manliness" (p.2).

Quick pharmaceutical fixes can treat this condition and prove men have the need for virility enhancing drugs such as Viagra. This sexual stimulus may cause men to ignore their decreased libido and the possibility of menopause. Driedger (1998) annotates that Viagra is undisputable proof that male menopause exists and is a widespread phenomenon. Over one million prescriptions were written for this potent drug within a two-month timeframe and 85% were for men over age 50. "They are voting with their pocketbooks to say, *I need something to bolster my potency*" (Driedger, 1998, p. 1). Denying menopause as a plausible problem, the drug Viagra has become popular because it stimulates men's libido. "The drug Viagra (sildenafil) has become the impotence drug of choice all over the world" (Rose, 2000, p. 108). The success of Viagra has other sex stimulating drugs becoming more available. "Shortly after Viagra was approved, news of other pills specifically designed to make it easier for men to have erections started to appear" (Spark, 2000, p. 135). Vasomax is only one sex-stimulating drug that came after Viagra. Since the inception of sex-stimulating drugs, men may feel validated in their belief and denial that male menopause does not exist. Being proactive about their health may decrease the need for men to take sex-stimulating drugs by learning more about testosterone replacement therapy.

The Implications of Hormone Replacement Therapy

Women appear to experience the same or similar physiological changes as men. Rose (2000) asserts, "male menopause has a much more gradual onset than female menopause" (p. 3). Women experience a decrease in estrogen as they age, according to

Rose (2000), "a woman's passage through middle age may be more noticeable because

her hormone levels may drop more rapidly" (p. 3); and "there is good evidence that

testosterone levels drop as a man ages" (Andropause, n.d., p. 3). The cardinal signs and

symptoms are irritability, decreased desire for sex, mood swings, weight gain, and

depression.

When men receive testosterone therapy, there is proof to show that "the

symptoms listed above will disappear" (Andropause, n.d., p. 4). However, there are some

exceptions with women because they usually complain of excruciating copulation, known

as dyspareunia. Dyspareunia is associated with the vaginal canal becoming dry due to the

decreasing levels of estrogen. "Beyond hot flashes, failing levels of estrogen may cause

vaginal dryness, leading to pain during intercourse" (Smolensky & Lamberg, 2000, p.

135). Additionally, similar to women, men may complain of fatigue that can negatively

affect sexual activity with their mates. "Men suffering from this 'syndrome' are said to

experience . . . fatigue and sluggishness, as well as a reduced interest in sex" (Wittmeier,

1999, p. 1). Decreased hormone levels also affect the ability of men and women to

procreate.

Women experiencing decreased hormone levels will eventually notice that they

no longer have menstrual cycles, which will mark the cessation of their childbearing

years. "She may have years of erratically fluctuating hormone levels, eventually followed

by a drop that causes her to stop having monthly cycles" (Rose, 2000, p. 3). Men,

however, may not notice a decrease in their testosterone levels right away. Much later in life, men will eventually notice decreasing testosterone levels as well as a decreasing

sperm count. Therefore, men's inability to impregnate a woman may not be seen until

many years after the first signs of andropause. "Although fertility may not be

dramatically affected, the hormonal changes that men go through from their thirties on

are significant" (Rose, 2000, p.3). With the current controversy regarding HRT, men and

women should explore all their options and discussed the best mode of treatment with

his/her physician.

Many men may become aware of a decreased interest in sexual intercourse, while

at the same time noticing that it is more difficult to maintain an erection. In addition, men

may complain of fatigue inside and outside the bedroom. "Testosterone can make a

difference in bed" (Lacayo & McLaughlin, 2000, p.1). Perhaps, the decreasing level of

testosterone is one of the worst aspects because it is associated with fatigue that may

cause men to be unable to please their partners sexually. Lacayo and McLaughlin (2000)

believe that testosterone produces "a roller coaster of emotional . . . effects, from a burst

of energy, snappishness, and libido . . . to fatigue" (p. 2). Declining estrogen and

testosterone levels in men and women are believed to cause many of the adverse side

effects that both genders experience during the perimenopausal and menopausal phases.

Researchers have long known that hormones, mainly estrogen and testosterone

play a significant role in balancing the affect of menopausal signs and symptoms.

However, there are still debates about the benefits and/or harm associated with hormone

replacement therapy. "The treatment is controversial. . . . Working out the right dosage

can be tricky" (Chaudhur, 2003, p.1). Testosterone replacement remains a highly contentious issue in the medical profession because of its associated hazards. "Risks surge of testosterone carries risk of liver problems, blood thickening, acne, and breast development and may accelerate growth of existing prostate" (Lacayo & McLaughlin, 2000, p.10). Some of the controversy surrounding hormone replacement is whether these hormones will stimulate sexual arousal, increase sexual pleasure, and restore individuals back to an active sex life. "Testosterone use still is controversial, both because testosterone may have unwanted side effects . . . . [And] it usually takes several weeks to show benefits" (Smolensky & Lamberg, 2000, p. 138). Because testosterone replacement is quite controversial, it is just as important to indicate some of its benefits. Mirkin (2002) states that testosterone injections can make older men with low blood levels of testosterone more interested in making love" (p. 1).

An outstanding benefit to testosterone replacement is that there is the possibility that a man can have a healthier libido and sex life. According to Lacayo and McLaughlin (2000), testosterone is responsible for increasing a man's libido or sex drive. Even with the risks involved, hormone replacement can be beneficial to men. Andropause (n.d.) verifies, "there is no doubt that the administration to [sic] testosterone to men with true testosterone deficiency . . . will improve their health and sense of well being" (p. 4). Furthermore, testosterone can slow down the aging process in men who fight against it and cause them to search for their second youth. "Swanton and Bryant (1998) state, "Testosterone therapy can improve the overall health and feeling of well-being of ageing men, improve sex drive, mental functions, and energy levels reducing the risk of cardiovascular disease" (p. 1). It is imperative that men speak with their physicians concerning the pros and cons of hormone replacement therapy or HRT.

There are concerns that arise with the use of testosterone, HRT; namely cancer and more specifically, prostate cancer. Men's Health (2004) cites Dr. Ballentine Carter saying, "testosterone replacement in older men increases the risk of prostate cancer" (p.1). Other than cancer, testosterone has been linked to various adverse side effects, which include "androgen-sensitive epilepsy, migraine, sleep apnea, polycythemia or fluid overload" (Mirkin, 2002, p. 1). Furthermore, some research has shown that with testosterone replacement therapy, some men may develop cardiovascular/heart problems.

A thorough physical examination should be conducted in an attempt to determine who may be at risk for taking hormone replacement therapy. In addition, a thorough examination will help determine who are the best candidates for this type of treatment. According to Mirkin (2003), there are two major concerns with testosterone replacement, which are the development of blood clots that can lead to a heart attack and the acceleration or worsening of a pre-existing problem such as prostate cancer.

CHAPTER THREE

The Methodology

Male menopause is a difficult subject to broach, especially with men. There may

be many ways to approach the study of this condition. Questions this study will explore

are: (a) how many men are aware of male menopause? (b) how many men do not regard

male menopause as reality? (c) men in denial about male menopause? (d) men willing to

consider the reality of this condition by displaying a willingness to address the problems

that male menopause may cause? (e) men aware at what age they are more likely to

experience menopause? (f) men ignorant about male menopause, or do they choose to be

in denial? This chapter further describes the research design used, identifies the

methodology, the population and sample chosen, and the instrumentation. The

methodology will also describe the data-collection method and data-analysis process.

Furthermore, Chapter Three will revisit the purpose of this study.

The overall purpose for this study is to determine the extent of men's lack of

knowledge or defiance about male menopause. The method describe in this chapter will

help determine the significance factors associated with testosterone and its association

with sexual activity. Because the incidence of male menopause is not widely known, this

author chose to study this disorder and its prevalence. This author used published research

to validate the existence of male menopause. Furthermore, this study examined, evaluated,

and explored ways of approaching the male population and how men should be educated

about this condition. Therefore, the impetus for managing menopause in men and women

is early detection, diagnosis, and treatment.

Conceptual Framework

The conceptual framework for which this topic was developed is based upon the negative connotation associated with male menopause. Diamond, J., Driedger, S. D., and Tan, R. S. all have existing theories that address (a) men's lack of understanding about andropause, (b) relevant predictors for diagnosing this condition, (c) the treatment modalities that men should consider, (d) the roles and responsibilities of healthcare providers for educating men about this condition, and (e) the age that men are more likely to begin experiencing signs and symptoms of andropause. These notable researchers, Diamond, J., Driedger, S. D., and Tan, R. S., as well as other authors, have written extensively about andropause and ways to educate and encourage men to seek more information about this condition.

Research Methodology

Using an independently designed questionnaire (survey) that is based on research literature, mainly Jed Diamond's (Appendix C), this writer surveyed approximately 200 men from the Detroit-Metropolitan Area. A letter was attached to the pre & posttest explaining the nature and purpose of the study. With the aid of an assistant, this author visited various sites to explain the survey and distribute them to the participants. This writer left the area, where the individuals were answering the surveys, to ensure that the participants did not feel uncomfortable or pressured. The assistant collected the surveys upon completion. The participants of the study, also, included healthcare professionals and physicians, to ascertain if there was any difference in their knowledge of male menopause.

The sampling method was a non-probability, convenience random sampling. Men were deliberately chosen relative to the characteristics needed to conduct the study. The characteristics will help to determine if there is any relevance regarding men's understanding about this condition, age, residency, employment, and if men have inquired about this condition with their physicians. A descriptive analysis incorporating frequency, ratio, and percentages, as defined below, aided in the analysis of the data obtained.

1. Frequency--by using an alpha scale of A-F, the author interpreted how frequently each item was answered. The relevance to how many times each item was answered determined if a man's age, beliefs, or knowledge base had an effect on how they view male menopause. Frequency was beneficial in showing, how many men knew about male menopause, what age men believed that they were most likely to experience menopause, if education had any significance to men's understanding or lack of understanding, and if younger men dismissed male menopause more often than older men.

2. Ratio- - was used in this study to measure and illustrate how many men agreed that male menopause existed and at what age were men at risk for developing this condition. Ratio helped pinpoint the age group of men that should be learning more about diagnosis and treatment.

3. Percentage- - was based on 100 percent total for every question. Each question is broken down into alpha categories, A-F; then, each item was weighed according to the responses received. From the results, a percentage rating was

assigned. Each item was weighed to determine if there was any validity to this researcher's belief that men deny or do not know that menopause exist.

Expected Findings

An Excel spreadsheet was used to tabulate the responses to each question. Each question had the same degree of weight (Appendix E). Using frequency, this author used the alpha scale of A through F, in the spreadsheet's cells; to interpret how many times each question had been answered. Based on the aforementioned 100 percent, a percentage rating was given to each question. A statistical correlation was done, focusing on questions 1 through 6, to discern if men know or do not know about male menopause. The end result was to find out, based on percentages, how many men were aware of male menopause and if other factors indicated that age, employment, or residency had anything to do with men's understanding or their lack of understanding. The expected response rate was 50% of the chosen population. After all of the statistics had been analyzed, this researcher either accepted or rejected the research question(s). The results of the analysis helped determine which men are most likely to experience menopause, so that interventions can begin early.

Research findings suggested that treatment should start as soon as possible, increasing the chance of favorable outcomes. However, one cannot be proactive without first understanding the causes of male menopause, ways to cope with it, and the fact that there is hope for continuing a healthy sex life. Research proposes preventative measures, ways to have a healthier sex life as men age, and decreasing the occurrence of impotency and loss of libido. This researcher purported that the expected findings would reveal that at least 50% of men from this study's chosen population had no idea that male menopause exists or men refuse to accept this concept. Doctors, nurses, and other healthcare providers can be instrumental in educating men about what they need to know concerning this condition.

Research findings further suggest that healthcare providers' should stay abreast of the progress being made in research relating to male menopause. The two areas that healthcare providers need to focus on are prevention and early diagnosis. Doctors and nurses should take the initiative to make appropriate recommendations and encourage men to live healthier lifestyles. Preventative measures could include monitoring abnormal signs and symptoms, being tested early, and reading the research literature available on male menopause. Implementing a survey, in the form of a questionnaire, helped discern, if men are aware that they are prone to this disorder. This survey could help determine if there is enough information available to educate men about menopause. Moreover, the design of this study was evaluated to determine what might be needed to assist men in preparing for a positive relationship with their health care practitioner.

Design of the Study

This study is a preordinate, qualitative (pre & posttest), as well as a cross-sectional descriptive design. According to Worthen, Sanders, and Fitzpatrick (1997) state that a "preordinate evaluation refers to evaluation studies that rely on prespecification, where inquiry tends to follow a prescribed plan and does not go beyond the predetermined issues and predefined problems" (p. 159). The author's pre-specifications were that each participant must be male, reside in the Detroit-Metropolitan Area, and be

willing to answer the survey questions honestly, and under their on volition.

A qualitative study "focuses on subjective data that is not easily coded into

numbers. The emphasis is on words and feelings rather than numbers. Qualitative

research tends to work with fewer subjects or respondents (cases) but analyses each case

to a deeper level" (Asia Market Research Dot Com, 2004, p. 1). Coding was used from

the questionnaire, in order to tally the survey questions and determine if men are either

aware or unaware of male menopause. The pre-test was used to analyze the

understanding that men have or do not have pertaining to male menopause. The post-test

provided the participants with vital information that could be used later, when these men

spoke with their physician. Gall, Gall, and Borg (2003) state that a cross-sectional study

collects "data at one point in time, but from samples that vary in age or developmental

stages" (p. 622). A descriptive study according to Gall, Gall, and Borg (2003), is "a type

of investigation that involves providing a detailed portrayal of one or more cases" (p.

623). These specific design types were chosen, to provide the author with more insight

into how many men from the study were unaware of male menopause versus those who

deny that male menopause exist. The eclectic approach was also used because many

approaches were needed to get answers about men and their understanding of menopause.

The eclectic approach includes objective, expertise, adversary, and participants.

1. The Objective approach looked at how the evaluator can achieve the

   objectives of the evaluation

2. The Adversary approach allowed this researcher to look at the pros and cons, while at the same time, not interjecting this researcher's own beliefs that could bias the evaluation process.

3. The Participant approach allowed the contributors and the researcher to become actively involved in the study. This approach could assist the participants in discovering new knowledge about male menopause and help the researcher evaluate the outcomes.

This design was chosen to examine the characteristics of approximately 200 men between the ages of 20-75. The intent of this study was to gain new insight into what men know or believe about male menopause.

Sample and Population

The participants selected were from a targeted population of approximately 200 men from 20-75 years of age. These individuals resided, predominately, in the Detroit-Metropolitan Area. The participants were randomly chosen based on age, economics, education, religious, and residency. These men were deliberately chosen relative to the above characteristics, which are needed to conduct the study.

Instrumentation

The survey was conducted from November 30, 2004 through January 8, 2005. Two-hundred questionnaires were distributed to men chosen for this study. The chosen geographical sites were in the Detroit-Metropolitan Area. There are 19 questions on this instrument that was authored by this researcher and was adapted from the researched literature. The majority of the questions were developed, based upon Jed Diamond's research, which can be retrieved from http://www.menalive.com. The post-test was

retrieved from Andropause.com. Twenty randomly chosen men participated in a pilot

survey, prior to the actual survey being distributed, which fit the afore-mentioned

characteristics. Both the pilot and the actual questionnaires addressed: (a) men's beliefs,

(b) if men get regular physical examinations, (c) residency, (d) age, (e) employment, (f)

and men's basic knowledge about male menopause.

   A letter accompanied the survey explaining, to the participants and the

participating sites, the nature of the study, and its purpose. Confidentiality was assured by

not having any traceable data on the survey that will identify the respondents.

Participation in the survey was solely voluntary with the option for the participants to

change their mind or withdraw from the study at anytime.

CHAPTER FOUR

Presentation and Analysis of the Data

One purpose for this study was to determine the extent of male ignorance or denial of male menopause. The study results suggested relevant predictors that could be used by health care professionals as criteria in the education and diagnosis of male menopause. Through research literature, the study investigated why this topic is not widely discussed in the medical community, and if early diagnosis could allow men to choose a treatment modality that is appropriate to their needs. The results of the study, which are described in the upcoming segment, will provide obvious and definitive information for healthcare providers to use when face with men who are potentially experiencing male menopause. As part of this study, the five research questions explored include the following:

1. How many men are aware of the concept of male menopause?

2. How many men do not regard male menopause as reality?

3. How many men know at what age they are more likely to experience menopause?

4. Of those men who accept the reality of this condition, how many are willing to address the problems that male menopause may cause.

5. What causes men to deny male menopause?

Descriptive Analysis of Statistics

From collected data, this author sought to discover the degree of understanding or lack of understanding that men have about male menopause. In addition, this study sought to quantify how many men deny male menopause and why. Therefore, a descriptive analysis incorporating frequency, ratio, and percentages, as defined below, aided in the analysis of the data obtained.

1. An alpha scale of A-F determined frequency. This researcher used the alpha scale to interpret how frequently each item was answered. The relevance to how many times each item was answered helped determine if a man's age, beliefs, or knowledge base had an effect on how they view male menopause. Frequency was beneficial in showing how many men knew about male menopause, what ages men believed that they were most likely to experience menopause, if education had any significance to men's understanding or lack of understanding, and if younger men dismissed this condition more often than older men.

2. Ratio (a scale of measure) was used in this study to illustrate how many men agreed that male menopause existed and at what age were men at risk for developing this condition. Ratio helped this researcher determine which age groups should be targeted to educate them more about diagnosis and treatment of male menopause.

3. Percentages were used, based on 100 percent total for each question on the survey. Every question was broken down into alpha categories, A-F; then each item was weighed according to the response received. From the results, a percentage rating was assigned. Each item was weighted to determine if men deny, do not understand, or do not know that menopause exist.

Implementation of the Study

Men who resided in the Detroit-Metropolitan Area participated in the study.

There were 200 questionnaires distributed to men who were 20-75 years of age. The

largest group of respondents was in the 61-75 year old age group. The participants were

randomly chosen predominantly based on gender; however, age, employment, and

residency were included to determine if there was a connection with any of the

aforementioned factors. The surveys were distributed November 1, 2004 through January

8, 2005. Although the amount of time needed to complete the surveys varied, on average,

the participants completed the surveys in less than 20 minutes.

Other Related Information

The male menopause questionnaire (pretest) primarily addressed if men were

aware of the term *male menopause* and if they believed that men were susceptible to this

condition. Men were asked about their understanding of the effects that male menopause

could have on them and if they knew about treatment modalities. The questionnaire asked

if men were aware what their testosterone levels meant and what was considered normal.

In addition, men were asked if they knew the age when men might be more susceptible to

male menopause. Another survey question asked if men visited their doctors regularly. In

addition, the survey sought to ascertain if the male participants broached the topic of

male menopause with other men and/or with their physicians (Appendix C).

The 10-question posttest questionnaire developed by John E. Morley, M. B., Ch,

titled *Do I Have Andropause* (Figure 4 and Appendix D), addressed typical signs and

symptoms that might indicate to men that they were experiencing andropause. The posttest intended use is to educate men about the signs and symptoms of male menopause and help men begin the dialogue with their physicians. The posttest could also be used as a self-assessment for men to help them understand the physiological and psychological changes they may be noticing. Men could have been experiencing psycho-physiological changes and not understood why these changes were occurring. Both the pre- and posttest, described in Chapter Three, could serve as educational tools to get men talking to their physicians and their spouses (Appendix C and D).

Pilot Survey

A pilot study was conducted by the instructor of the men at a local community college. The men from the pilot study were enrolled in a heating, ventilation, and air-conditioning program (HVAC). Twenty surveys (pretest) were given to the male students' instructor and then distributed to the class yet there were 15 respondents. In order to ensure the subjects confidentiality, this researcher was not in the room at the time the surveys were being completed. The fifteen voluntary participants were from the ages of 20 to 60 years of age. Ten men were 20 to 30 years of age, two men were 31-40 years of age, two men were 41-50 years of age, and one man was in the age group of 51-60.

The pilot study results included the following: (a) some men had never heard of the term male menopause; (b) not all men believed they could experience male menopause; (c) four men did not think that they needed to address menopause; (d) four men stated that they are not sure that they will experience male menopause; and (e) six men stated that they are not ready to address this condition. The comments documented from the pilot study may be attributed to the ages of the men, being 20 to 30 years of age.

According to research, the average age for male menopause is 40. "The most common problem associated with male menopause is depression which is closely related to impotence and problems with male sexuality . . . . 40% of men in their 40s . . . will [experience] male menopause" (Diamond, 2003, p. 1). The results of the pilot pretest are delineated below in Table 1 and Figure 3. The actual questions from the survey can be found in Appendix C.

Table 1

An Analysis of the Pilot Study Results

Question No.	A Yes	B No	C	D	E	Totals	Question No.	%A	%B	%C	%D	%E
#1	3	12				15	#1	20.0%	80.0%	0.0%	0.0%	0.0%
#2	3	12				15	#2	20.0%	80.0%	0.0%	0.0%	0.0%
#3	10	0	1	4		15	#3	66.7%	0.0%	6.7%	26.7%	0.0%
#4	1	13	1			15	#4	6.7%	86.7%	6.7%	0.0%	0.0%
#5	15	0	0	0		15	#5	100.0%	0.0%	0.0%	0.0%	0.0%
#6	1	3	10	1		15	#6	6.7%	20.0%	66.7%	6.7%	0.0%
#7	14	1				15	#7	93.3%	6.7%	0.0%	0.0%	0.0%
#8	10	2	2	1	0	15	#8	66.7%	13.3%	13.3%	6.7%	0.0%
#9	1	5	9			15	#9	6.7%	33.3%	60.0%	0.0%	0.0%
#10	0	15	0			15	#10	0.0%	100.0%	0.0%	0.0%	0.0%
#11	0	15				15	#11	0.0%	100.0%	0.0%	0.0%	0.0%
#12	0	0	0	15	0	15	#12	0.0%	0.0%	0.0%	100.0%	0.0%
#13	4	5	2	4		15	#13	26.7%	33.3%	13.3%	26.7%	0.0%
#14	0	15				15	#14	0.0%	100.0%	0.0%	0.0%	0.0%
#15	0	15				15	#15	0.0%	100.0%	0.0%	0.0%	0.0%
#16	9	6				15	#16	60.0%	40.0%	0.0%	0.0%	0.0%
#17	11	4				15	#17	73.3%	26.7%	0.0%	0.0%	0.0%
#18	0	0				0	#18	0.0%	0.0%	0.0%	0.0%	0.0%
#19	14	1				15	#19	93.3%	6.7%	0.0%	0.0%	0.0%

The survey asked specific questions to ascertain to what level the men were at in their acceptance of male menopause or if they were willing to begin dialogue related to this topic. The detailed results are as follows for each response above and are reflective of each numbered item preceding:

1. Eighty percent of the men indicated that they were aware of the term male menopause.

2. Eighty percent of the male respondent believed that it is *possible* for men to experience male menopause.

3. Conversely, close to 67% of the respondents indicated that male menopause does not exist.

4. Close to 87% percent of the men believed that there was no treatment for this disorder, 6.7% believed male menopause could be treated, and 6.7% was unsure.

5. One hundred percent of the respondents indicated that surgery is the treatment modality for male menopause.

6. Approximately 7% believed that men are susceptible to male menopause between the ages of 20-38, 20% believed men were more susceptible after age 39, 66.7%, indicated that men do not experience menopause, and 6.7% were not sure.

7. Greater than ninety-three percent responded that they would like to learn more about this condition, 6.7% responded no to learning more about male menopause.

8. The respondents' age ranges were 66.7% were 20-30 years of age, 13.3% were 31-40 and 41-50 years of age, respectively, 6.7% were 51-70 years of age, and 0% was greater than 61 years old.

9. Sixty percent resided in suburban areas of the Detroit-Metropolitan Area, while 33.3% resided in the city and 6.7% resided in rural areas.

10. One Hundred percent of the respondents were students.

11. None of the respondents has seen a doctor to have their testosterone levels drawn.

12. None of the respondents had any idea what their testosterone levels were.

13. The responses indicated that 26.7% had a doctor's visit within the last 3 months (of the time they had taken the survey), 33.3% visited the doctor within one year, 13.3% indicated that their last doctor's visit was longer than one year, and 26.7% did not go to the doctor on a regular basis.

14. When asked if the participants' doctors discussed male menopause, 100% answered no.

15. When the participants were asked if they inquired of their doctors about male menopause, 100%, responded no also.

16. Sixty percent of the respondents' physicians were male and 40% were female.

17. Greater than 73% indicated that they are more likely to inquire about male menopause, since taking this questionnaire.

18. Question number 18 was an essay question that asked if the respondents answered no to the previous question (#17). The responses varied from not needing to worry about male menopause, the majority of the respondents were 20-30 years of age, to some participants not being sure that they will ever experience male menopause.

19. After completing this questionnaire, 93.3% indicated that they felt more

prepared to ask their physicians about male menopause.

Figure 3

This following graph will provide visual information for the preceding table.

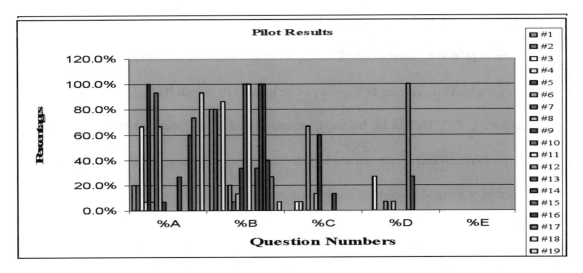

An Analysis of the Pretest Responses

This author set out to investigate if at least 50% of the participants were in denial

about male menopause. Furthermore, this study intended to identify the percentage of

males who were unaware of male menopause. The renowned authors and researchers on

this topic are Diamond, J., Driedger, S. D., and Tan, R. S., who suggested that there was a

link to male menopause and declining testosterone levels. Furthermore, the

aforementioned authors support the belief that diagnosis and treatment is significant to

alleviating symptoms and providing a healthier sex life. Therefore, this author conducted

a study that analyzed to what extent past research imitated real life.

There were 200 surveys (pretest) distributed, with 104 (52%) respondents

(Appendix C). The research questions one through five, which are found in Chapter One and in the beginning of this chapter, reflect the responses to questions 1, 2, 6, 15, and 18, respectively (Appendix E). The selected questions, listed above, were germane to this study because it assisted in identifying if men have some knowledge about male menopause and if men are discussing this topic with their primary care physicians. Chapter One delineated the findings from the data. Table 2, below, links the significant responses related to questions 1, 2, 6, 15, and 18 of the study and the research questions from Chapter One. The entire survey can be located in Appendix C. In the responses to questions 1, 2, 6, 15, and 18, below, frequency aided in interpreting how often each item was answered. Ratio illustrated the targeted age groups of the study. Additionally, the percentages assigned weight to each question.

Table 2

An Analysis of the Five Research Questions and Survey Responses

Question Numbers	A	B	C	D	E	F
1. Are you aware of the term male menopause?	47 (45.2%) Yes	57 (54.8%) No	N/A	N/A	N/A	N/A
2. Do you believe men can acquire male menopause?	35 (33.7%) Yes	14 (13.5%) No	55 (52.9%) Unsure	N/A	N/A	N/A
6. What age do you think men are more susceptible to male menopause?	2 (1.9%) 20-30 years of age	39 (37.5%) After age 39	10 (9.6%) Men do not experience male menopause	53 (51%) Unsure	N/A	N/A
15. Did you ask your physician about male menopause?	4 (3.8%) Yes	92 (88.5%) No	8 (7.7%) No response	N/A	N/A	N/A
18. Briefly explain why you are less likely to inquire about male menopause.	76 (73.1%) Answered yes to number 17.	28 (26.9%) Answered no to number 17, with explanation	N/A	N/A	N/A	N/A

The responses to number 18 asked men if they were more likely to inquire about male menopause with their physicians or not (Appendix C). Some of the male participants annotated their thoughts about male menopause as it related to them specifically. The men's responses included these short statements:

1. "I never asked."

2. "Don't feel affected by it now."

3. "No need."

4. "Doesn't interest me."

5. "I feel satisfied with my health."

6. "Why and what is it?"

7. "Not interested."

8. "I don't think it affects me."

9. "Maybe, I am of the age when it occurs."

10. Four men stated, "I'm too young."

11. "Not concerned."

12. "It will not affect me for awhile."

13. "I don't care about this."

14. "Because it is common for men 40 and older and that is not me."

15. "I don't feel the need to know."

16. "Hopefully, it does not concern me."

17. "I do not believe I will ever deal with it."

18. "I feel I am too young to have it apply."

19. "It does not concern me yet."

20. "So far, so good."

21. "No complaints."

22. "I don't believe men get it."

23. "It does not exist."

In Chapter One, the expected number of responses was projected to be 50% of the chosen population. There were 52%, of the predicted 50%, that responded to this survey. Therefore, this author met the projected response rate for this survey. The results collected from the surveys, using frequency, ratio, and percentages, answered the aforementioned research questions (Table 2, Appendix E, and F).

Posttest Questionnaire Results

The posttest (Appendix D) mainly focused on men's psychological and physiological experiences that could be indicative of male menopause. By answering the 10 questions on the survey, men could gain more insight about the changes that may be occurring. Furthermore, the design of the posttest was to assist men in gaining knowledge as well as educate them how better to talk with their physicians about this condition. The entire set of results from the posttest is located in Appendix F. The condensed results in Tables 2 and 3, above, can be viewed in their entirety (Appendix E & F). Both questionnaires (pre- and posttest) are also available in its entirety in Appendix C and Appendix D. Interestingly, Table 3 illustrated that the majority of men from the study denied a decrease in libido and erectile strength, two main indicators associated with male menopause.

Table 3

An Analysis of How Men Perceived Their Libido and Erectile Function

Question Numbers	Yes	No
3. Do you have a decrease in your sex drive (libido)?	29 (31.9%)	59 (64.8%)
9. Are your erections less strong?	32 (35.2%)	59 (64.8%)

Summary

This chapter presented the results of the statistical analysis from the pre- and posttest scores. The method used was non-probability, convenience random sampling because the male participants were deliberately chosen relative to the characteristics needed to conduct the study. The participants had to be males between the ages of 20 to 75. An Excel spreadsheet was used to compile the data looking at frequency, ratio, and percentages. The five research questions were answered as follows:

1. How many men are aware of the concept of male menopause? Approximately, 45% are aware, while 54.8% were not (pretest question number 1).

2. How many men do not regard male menopause as reality? Thirty-Three percent did not believe that male menopause exists (number 2 of pretest), 13.5% did not believe male menopause exists, and 52.9% indicated that they were unsure.

3. How many men know at what age they are more likely to experience menopause? Thirty-Seven and one-half percent believed men could experience this condition after the age of 39, which is consisted with the literature, refer to pretest question number 6).

4. Of those men who accept the reality of this condition, how many were willing to address the potential problems that male menopause could cause. Number 15 of the pretest addressed if men have talked with their doctors about male menopause and 88.5% indicated that they have not.

5. What causes men to deny male menopause? On the pretest, men wrote down their answers to why they are less likely to inquire about male menopause. The responses are delineated above; refer to the responses following Table 2 in this chapter.

Table 3 results focused on two questions from the posttest. Number 3 asked the respondents, did they have a decrease in their sex drive (libido)? Out of 100%, nearly 65% answered no. Number 9 asked the male participants if their erections were less strong and 64.7% responded no. Based on Table 2 and 3's responses, this researcher is reminded of one of the limitations from this study that was indicated in Chapter Two. It was this researcher contention that because of the sensitive nature of this topic, the participants may not answer the questions truthfully. Therefore, additional research needs to be done to ascertain if this study's results can be duplicated netting the same of similar results. Furthermore, educating men about male menopause may remove the stigma that it is a female condition instead of a natural transition of life and aging for both genders.

CHAPTER FIVE

Summary, Conclusions, Implications, and Recommendations

This study was undertaken primarily to determine whether men were aware that

male menopause existed, also known as andropause or male climacteric. The first three

research questions specifically addressed men's awareness or lack of awareness of male

menopause. They were: (a) how many men are aware of the concept of male menopause,

(b) how many men do not regard male menopause as reality, and (c) what causes men to

deny male menopause. The fourth question specifically addressed, of those men who

accept the reality of this condition, how many are willing to address the potential

problems that male menopause may cause. The fifth and final question mainly addressed

how many men know at what age they are more susceptible to experiencing menopause?

Chapter Five will summarize the study, draw conclusions from the study, make

recommendations, and include this researchers implications pertaining to the study.

Summary of the Study

This research literature has shown that male climacteric is as real for men as it is

for women. Rose (2000) asserts, "the men being studied actually experience some of the

same symptoms women experience at menopause" (p. 4). Chapter Two delineates the

signs and symptoms of male and female menopause and their similarities. Moreover,

more research is needed to explore how best to educate men about this natural biological

change of life. Spark (2000) suggests that this is "a natural consequence of advancing

age" (p. 366). Furthermore, men need to become familiarized with the signs and symptoms that will prompt them to seek health care professionals for proper screening, diagnosis, and treatment. According to Driedger (1998), many men dismiss the symptoms like mood swings, irritability, and decreased sexual desire. Many men may believe that the symptoms are not associated with male menopause and would rather not discuss it.

Summary of the finding Related to the Conclusion

Earlier in the study, male menopause was defined, along with its associated terminology. This study further described how the decline in testosterone plays a significant role in the diagnostic process and the effects testosterone has on libido. Furthermore, this study proposed through analysis of previously studied and reported upon data that the change of life in men and male midlife crisis occurs when men begin to experience male climacteric. Moreover, this study discussed what previous literature reports about the similarities and differences between male and female climacteric. In addition, the literature evaluated the knowledge and emotion that men have pertaining to male menopause. Finally, based upon reported literature, this study defended the realism that men and women experience the same and/or similar signs and symptoms associated with menopause.

The literature has made it clear that men do not take menopause as seriously as they should; this is just one of the reasons why health practitioners need to explore ways to educate men about the reality of male menopause. "Many have questioned whether the male menopause is more myth than reality" (Tan, 2001, p. 10). The literature suggests areas that health practitioners should focus on, when educating men about male menopause and what physical changes occur and how these changes are similar to female menopause. The design of the posttest was incorporated in this study to assist men in gaining knowledge, while at the same time preparing them how better to talk with their physicians about this condition. The survey results indicated that more than 54% of men were unaware of male menopause (Chapter Four, Table 2).

Conclusions

As previously mentioned, some men are more apt to believe that menopause happens only to women because male menopause is a controversial phenomenon. Spark (2000) states that some men are very "ardent in insisting that there is no evidence for the existence of either a male climacteric or a male menopause" (p. 363). It is of paramount importance that men come to understand that menopause is not only a female concern. More importantly, men should be made aware that menopause is a natural phase of life. Yet, men struggle with accepting menopause as their reality. Ironically, research has shown that female menopause is a very familiar concept, whereas, male menopause is not mainly because female menopause has been studied in more depth. "Andropause in men is relatively uncommon, compared to . . . menopause in women" (Andropause, n.d., p. 1).

Based on the ongoing debate about the validity of male menopause, with men and their physicians, diagnosis and treatment could be delayed. Schieszer (2004) writes about Dave O'Neal, a 47-year-old man who experienced serious health problems that continued until he finally found a physician that properly diagnosed him with andropause. O'Neal began receiving testosterone injections twice a month for five years without the reoccurrence of the symptoms he had experienced associated with male menopause and depression.

Recommendations

The information presented in this study corroborates that male menopause is a controversial topic. To dispel the controversy, a collaborative effort among men, women, health care professionals, and the media is needed by bringing more awareness to this condition. Because of the debate surrounding the reality of male menopause in relation to female menopause, health care professionals should continue the dialogue with men to dispel the belief that menopause only affect women. Furthermore, physicians need to find alternative methods, other than Viagra, to address men's problems with decreased libido.

Early detection and treatment are two methods that physicians should stress to men in order to ward-off any sexual concerns that may arise later. For these reasons, health care providers, various organizations, authors, and society will need to continue the mission to educate men about the signs and symptoms for this disorder. Schieszer (2004) writes that Dr. John Morley "is calling on the Federal Government to fund a major study" (p. 2).

Another approach could be male seminars about male menopause, which could be an effective way to assist those men that are more accepting of male menopause and get them talking about this phenomenon, while offering support to those men having a difficult time accepting this condition. Men could talk with men experiencing signs and symptoms of menopause. Support groups will help men learn that they are not alone. Furthermore, men could benefit from printed literature pertaining to male menopause in an attempt to encourage them to consider the pros and cons about male menopause.

The media's role has changed, over the years, by becoming an added resource for disseminating information to a broader audience. In doing so, the negative social stigma has been lifting. More men are learning that it is no longer taboo to talk about male menopause. The media should continue to inform men about male menopause and encourage men to see their physicians early for screening. Moreover, the media can inform men about the psychological and physiological signs and symptoms so that they are prepared to open up dialogue with their physicians and other men. Physicians, healthcare providers, and the media's overall goal should be to decrease anxiety and increase awareness.

The research literature has clearly proven that male menopause exists and that men are diagnosed with male menopause at a higher rate today than in the past. According to Schieszer (2004), "men who are middle-aged today will live well into their 80s and 90s and need to be concerned about this issue" (p. 4). However, even with documented cases of male menopause, viropause, male climacteric, or andropause it remains a source of contention for many men. The research literature validate that men are more informed about changes that women go through than changes that men go though themselves. Female menopause is more familiar and accepting for men than male menopause. "Men who have watched this whole process, or who are in the middle of helping a loved one through it, may have breathed a sigh of relief that they don't have to go through it themselves" (Rose, 2000, p.3).

Because many men are refusing to consider male menopause as a viable transition through the aging process, it becomes quite difficult to educate them about this phenomenon. Therefore, it is a major concern that many men do not accept or do not understand the impact this condition can have on them physiologically and psychologically. It is apparent from reading the research literature that countless men are in denial about the reality of male climacteric. The research literature further strengthens the argument that men need to be better educated about this condition.

With all of the ambiguity surrounding menopause and the fact that men are very apprehensive about accepting the actuality of male menopause, it is apparent that men are putting themselves more at risk by not addressing their sexual concerns. Seeking early diagnosis, counseling, and treatment can decrease any adverse risk to men's health and sexual prowess. Men should address any issues associated with andropause early. Armed with this awareness and understanding their family relationships could conceivably be saved or enhanced.

As discussed in Chapter Two, research has shown that long-term marriages have ended for seemingly unknown reasons. More men should take a simple blood test to help determine if they are entering menopause. This diagnosis could offer reasonable treatment options that can reintroduce physiological and psychological balance. Addressing the signs and symptoms early could be beneficial in allaying fears and enhancing men's libido. Proper treatment can decrease the chance of men "straying away", destroying their relationships and that of their families. An additional concern for men could be attributed to their fear of having to address end-of-life issues.

End-of-life issues can be addressed, if men decide early to obtain information that would explain and clarify their concerns. Becoming better educated could relieve some of the stress associated with andropause and concerns with death and dying. It appears that men are fighting to remain *men* until the end. Maintaining their manhood seems to be paramount on the list of concerns pertaining to the whole debate concerning male menopause. Needless to say, more information needs to be made available and the issue of male menopause needs to be openly discussed.

It is vitally importance that men consult their primary physicians and other health professionals for early screening. More importantly, the whole issue of male menopause has to be brought to the attention of the entire health care community as well as the public. Society, especially men, should be educated about the implications of male menopause. As with most health concerns, early treatment and prevention are the best ways to tackle any health problems, including male menopause.

Discussion and Implications

While conducting this study, this writer went a step further and spoke with a few male physicians to ascertain if they (a) believe male menopause exists, (b) talk with their male clients about the implications of male menopause, and (c) routinely monitor men's testosterone levels to obtain a baseline for follow-up care. From the conversations with the aforementioned physicians, this author determined that these physicians were not vested in the ideology that male menopause is as significant as female menopause. The doctors who participated in the study indicated that they do not routinely monitor testosterone levels or address male menopause with their male patients. The doctors' responses were evident in the participants' responses, numbers 11, 12, 14, 15, and 16 on the survey (Appendix C).

Limitations and Delimitations

The overall objective of this study was to explore how research literature described menopause as a natural maturation process of the life cycle. Limitation with this methodology, compared to other studies, identified a need for future quantitative research and theory testing. Further research can evaluate and validate the leading researchers' reputation to determine how men are educated about male menopause and why menopause is mainly viewed as a female disease. This author used historical data, based on information found in the research literature. As previously mentioned, the leading research conducted on male menopause has been done by Diamond, J., Driedger, S. D., and Tan, R. S. The sample and population used in this study suggested that men did not know or did not have a good grasp about male menopause. This study further suggested that many men did not believe that male menopause exists (80%). However, as stated earlier, the literature showed that men were more accepting of female menopause. Therefore, this study has shown that more work still needs to be done in order to educate men about male menopause. In doing so, perhaps men will be convinced that male menopause is a condition that they will have to address as they age.

References

Ahlborg, H. G. (2003). Changes in bone mass and skeletal structure in the

    postmenopausal period [Electronic version]. *Heath Sciences, Medicine And*

    Surgery; Health Sciences, Obstetrics And Gynecology; Health Sciences, Human

    Development. Retrieved April 07, 2004 from http:// wwwlib.umi.com/

    dissertations/fullcit/f316657.

Andropause. (n.d.). Retrieved May 13, 2004 from http://www.midlife-

    passage.com/hormones.htm.

Andropause. *Getting older is natural. Feeling older is optional.* (n.d.). Retrieved August

    18, 2004, from http://www.andropause.com.

Asia Market Research Dot Com. (2004). Qualitative Research [Electronic Version].

    Retrieved on August 28, 2004 from http://www.asiamarketresearch.com/

    glossary/qualitative-research.htm.

Axley, L. B. (2003). Midlife women making decisions about menopause symptoms

    [Electronic version]. *Health Sciences, Nursing.* Retrieved April 07, 2004 from

    http://wwwlib.umi.com/dissertations/fullcit/3085393.

Barrett-Conner, E., Won Muhlen, D. G., & Kritz-Silverstein, D. (1999, February).

    Bioavailability testosterone and depressed mood in older men: the Rancho

    Bernardo Study [Electronic version]. *ZRT Laboratory.* Retrieved April 12, 2004

    from http://www.salivatest.com/store/bhrt_testosterone.html.

Chase, M. (1998, February 2). Aging men lose testosterone, but it isn't male menopause

[Electronic version]. *Wall Street Journal*. Retrieved April 07, 2004 from

http://library.capella.edu:2226/pqdweb?index.

Chaudhuri, A. (2003, November 02). Testosterone is boosting women's staying power in

the boardroom and the bedroom [Electronic version]. *Library Journal*. Retrieved

April 04, 2004 from http://library.capella.edu:2241/universe/document?_m.

Cohen, S. (2003, November 11). Menopause occurs in men, too [Electronic version].

Life-Health. Retrieved April 04, 2004 from http:// library.capella.edu:2241/

universe/document?_m.

Diamond, J. (2003). Male menopause: Men and depression [Electronic version].

Retrieved May 13, 2004 from http:// www.healthyplace.com/Communities/

Depression/men/asp.

Diamond, J. (2004). What do women want to know about male menopause? A chat with

Jed at the Power-Surge Web Site [Electronic version]. Retrieved October 6, 2004

from http://www.menalive.com/powersurgechat.htm.

Driedger, S. D. (1998, June 08). 'Mind over manliness' [Electronic version]. *Maclean's*.

Retrieved April 07, 2004 from http://library.capella.edu:2226/pqdweb?index.

Eastman, P. (2004, February). Real men see doctors. *AARP Bulletin*, p.16.

Foresta, C., Caretta, N., & Rossato, M. (2003, September). Erectile function in elderly:

role of androgens [Electronic version]. *Aging Male*. Retrieved April 12, 2004

from http://proquest.umi.com/pqdlink?index=5&did=000000487423521&

SrchMode=3

Fatusi, A. O., Ljadunola, K. T., Ojofeitimi, E. O., et al. (2003, June). Assessment of Andropause awareness and erectile dysfunction among married men in Ile-Ife, Nigeria [Electronic version]. *Aging Male*. Retrieved April 12, 2004 from http://proquest.umi.com/pqdlink?index=2&did=000000395360151&SrchMode=3

Gall, M. D., Gall, J. P., & Borg, W. R. (2003). *Educational research: an introduction* (Seventh Edition). Boston: Allyn and Bacon.

Gearon, C. J. (2004). Dealing with male menopause [Electronic version]. *Discovery Health Channel*. Retrieved August 16, 2004 from http://health.discovery.com/ centers/mens/andropause/andropause.html

Goodwin, J. S. (2001, April 28). Narcissus drowned [Electronic version]. *Lancet*. Retrieved April 04, 2004 from http://library.capella.edu:2226/pqdweb?index

Gould, D. C., Petty, R. & Jacobs, H. S. (2003). For and against: The male menopause— does it exist. *British Medical Journal, 320,858-61*.

Gruenewald, D. A. & Matsumoto, A. M. (2003, January). Testosterone supplementation therapy for older men: Potential benefits and risks [Electronic version]. *Journal of the American Geriatrics Society*. Retrieved April 10, 2004 from http://search.epnet.com/direct.asp?an=8875369&db=aph&loginpage=1

Hodges, F. M. (2003, March). The penalties of passion and desire: Love and the aging male in early 20th-century film [Electronic version]. *Aging Male*. Retrieved April 12, 2004 from http://proquest.umi.com/pqdlink?index=5&did=000000350190381 & SrchMode=3

Hollander, E. (2003, August). Hypogandadism: Psychiatric implications of male menopause [Electronic version]. *Psychiatric Annals*. Retrieved April 07, 2004 from http://library.capella.edu:2226/pqdweb?index

Hollander, E. & Samons, D. M. (2003, August). Male menopause: An unexplored area of men's health [Electronic version]. *Psychiatric Annals*. Retrieved April 07, 2004 from http://library.capella.edu:2226/pqdweb?index

Ian, P. (2003, January 23). The male menopause possible causes, symptoms and treatment [Electronic version]. *British Journal of Nursing*. Retrieved April 10, 2004 from http://search.epnet.com/direct.asp? an=9017241&db=aph&loginpage= loginin.a.

Is it Andropause? (n.d.). *Postgraduate medicine*. Retrieved April 04, 2004 from http://library.capella.edu:2144/citation.asp?tb=1.

Isaac, P. E. (2002, Winter). Male menopause and men of African descent [Electronic version]. *Journal of African American* Men. Retrieved April 05, 2004 from http://by2fd.bay.hotmail.msn.com/cgi-bin/getmsg?curmbox= F000000001&a =86426f034ae.

Kessenrich, C. R. (2000, August). Inevitable Menopause. *Nursing Profile Magazine*.

Lacayo, R. & McLaughlin, L. (2000, April 04). Are you man enough [Electronic version]? *Men – Physiology*. Retrieved April 10, 2004 from http://search.epnet.com/direct.asp?an=2992861&db=aph&loginpage=1.

LeShan, E. (1973). *The wonderful crisis of middle age*. New York: David McKay Company, INC.

Lord, D. C. (2000, October 15). Surviving male menopause: A guide for women and men [Electronic version]. *Library Journal*. Retrieved April 07, 2004 from http://library.capella.edu:2226/pqdweb?index.

Luboshitzky, R., Shen-Orr, Z., & Herer, P. (2003, September). Middle-aged men secrete less testosterone at night than young healthy men [Electronic version]. *Aging Male*. Retrieved April 12, 2004 from http://proquest.umi.com /pqdlink?index= 8&did=000000487423531&SrchMode.

Mayer, N. (1978). *The male mid-life crisis: Fresh starts after 40*. New York: Doubleday & Company, Inc.

McCarthy, B. & McCarthy, E. (1998). *Male sexual awareness: Increasing sexual satisfaction (Revised ed.)*. New York: Carroll & Graf Publishers, INC.

Midlife Men: (ages 40 to 60). (2000, April). *Natural Health Ltd*. Retrieved April 06, 2004 from http://www.capella/johnshopkinsuniversity.

Mirkin, G. (2002, March). Testosterone replacement for older men [Electronic version]? *Journal of Psychiatry*. Retrieved April 12, 2004 from http://www.drmirkin.com/ men/M227.html.

Morley, J. E. (2002). Diagnosis: Do I have andropause [Electronic version]? *Andropause.com*. Retrieved August 18, 2004 from http://www.andropause.com/ diagnosis/quiz.asp.

Munoz, S. S. (2003, November 13). Men shouldn't use testosterone to ward off aging, panel warns [Electronic version]. *Wall Street Journal*. Retrieved April 07, 2004 from http://library.capella.edu:2226/pqdweb?index.

Newman, L. (1996, October). Will testosterone replacement turn back clock for aging

men [Electronic version]? *Urology Times.* Retrieved April 05, 2004 from

http://library.capella.edu:2144/citation.asp?tb=1.

Physiologic factors: Is Andropause the "male menopause"? (2004, January).

Postgraduate medicine. Retrieved April 04, 2004 from

http://library.capella.edu:2241/universe/document?_m.

Papalia, D. E., Olds, S. W., & Feldman, R. D. (2001). *Human development (8th ed.).*

Boston: McGraw Hill.

Perry, A. (2001). *A comprehensive, up-to-date guidebook for achieving optimal health*

and fitness: American Medical Association Complete Guide – Men's health. New

York: John Wiley & Sons, Inc.

Puskar, J. (n.d.). Are you in male menopause? *Natural Health Ltd.* Retrieved April 06,

2004 from http://www.capella/johnshopkinsuniversity.

Rose, M. R. (2000). *A woman's guide to male menopause: Real solutions for helping him*

maintain vitality and virility. Los Angeles: Keats Publishing.

Schieszer, J. (2004). Male menopause out of the closet: More men being treated as

concerns about condition grow. *MSNBC's Guide To Men's Sexual Health.*

Retrieved May 13, 2004 from http://msnbc.msn.com/id/3543479.

Six Degrees of Separation. (n.d.). Retrieved December 9, 2004, from

http://www.aries.mos.org/six degrees.

Smolensky, M. & Lamberg, L. (2000). *The body clock: Guide to better health.* New

York: Henry Holt & Company.

Spark, R. F.   (2000). *Sexual health for men: The complete guide.* Massachusetts: Perseus

    Publishing.

Steidle, C. (2004). Andropause: An introduction [Electronic version]. *Seekwellness.*

    Retrieved December 9, 2004, from http://www.seekwellness.com/andropause.

Stuttaford, G., Simson, M., & Zaleski, J. (1997, August 04). Male menopause [Electronic

    version]. *Publishers Weekly.* Retrieved April 07, 2004 from

    http://library.capella.edu:2226/pqdweb?index.

Swanton, J. (1998, April 01). The testosterone syndrome: The critical factor for energy,

    health, & sexuality; reversing the male menopause [Electronic version]. *Library*

    Journal. Retrieved April 07, 2004 from http://library.capella.edu:2226/

    pqdweb?index.

Swanton, J. & Eric, B. (1998, April 01). The testosterone syndrome: The critical factor

    for energy, health, & sexuality; reversing the male menopause [Electronic

    version]. *Science & Technology.* Retrieved April 05, 2004 from

    http://library.capella.edu:2144/citation.asp?tb=1.

Tan, R. S. (2004, January). Is it andropause [Electronic version]? *Postgraduate Medicine.*

    Retrieved April 04, 2004 from http://library.capella.edu:2144/citation.asp?tb=1.

Tan, R. S. (2001). *The andropause mystery: Unraveling truths about male menopause.*

    Houston, Texas: AMRED Publishing.

Thomas, C. L. (1997). *Taber's Cyclopedic Medical Dictionary* (18 ed.). Philadelphia: F.

    A. Davis Company.

Wittmeir, C. (1999, April 26). Turn on, tune in, wake up: Boomers who idolized sexual

potency are suffering an identity crisis [Electronic version]. *Newsmagazine*

Retrieved April 07, 2004 from http://library.capella.edu:2226/pqdweb?index.

Worthen, B., Sanders, J., & Fitzpatrick, J. (1997). *Program evaluation: Alternative*

approaches and practical guidelines (2nd ed.). White Plains, NY: Sage.

APPENDIX A

A depiction of the male sex-organs, including the testes. Taber's Cyclopedic Medical

Dictionary, Vol. 18, pages 1433.

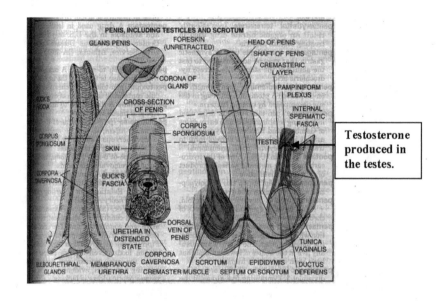

APPENDIX B

A depiction of the interstitial cells of the testes that is responsible for hormone production

in men. Retrieved from Taber's Cyclopedic Medical Dictionary, Vol. 18, page 1927.

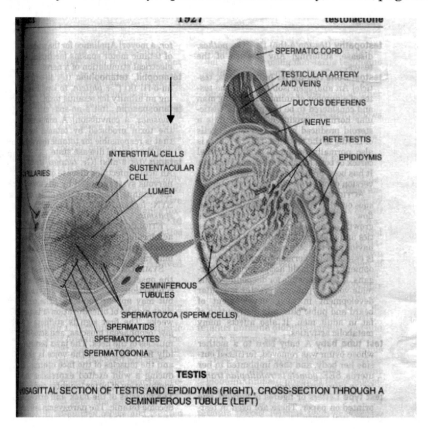

APPENDIX C
Male Menopause
This is a Confidential Voluntary Questionnaire-Pretest

Please read each question carefully and circle your answer. Choose only one response per question.

1.) Are you aware of the term "**male** menopause"?
    A.) Yes
    B.) No

2.) Do you believe men can acquire male menopause?
    A.) Yes
    B.) No
    C.) Unsure

3.) What is your understanding about the effects of male menopause?
    A.) It does not exist
    B.) It affects libido (sex drive)
    C.) I am not sure
    D.) Menopause only occurs with women

4.) To your knowledge, is there any treatment?
    A.) Yes
    B.) No
    C.) Unsure

5.) If you answered yes to number 4, what do you believe the treatment to be?
    A.) Surgery
    B.) Hormone replacement therapy
    C.) Oral medication
    D.) All of the above

6.) What age do you think men are more susceptible to male menopause?
    A.) Between 20-38
    B.) After the age of 39
    C.) Men do not experience menopause
    D.) I am not sure

7.) Would you like to learn more about male menopause?
    A.) Yes
    B.) No

8.) What is your age range?
    A.) 20-30
    B.) 31-40
    C.) 41-50
    D.) 51-60
    E.) 61-75

9.) What area do you reside in?
    A.) Rural (country)
    B.) Urban (city)

C.) Suburban
D.) Other(please specify) _____
10.) List your job title:
    A.) Retired
    B.) Student
    C.) Unemployed
    D.) Other (please specify) _____
11.) Have you seen a doctor to have your testosterone levels drawn?
    A.) Yes
    B.) No
12.) What was your testosterone level?
    A.) 800-1000
    B.) 600-999
    C.) 300-599
    D.) unknown
13.) When was your last doctor visit?
    A.) Within last 3 months
    B.) One year ago
    C.) Longer than one year
    D.) I do not go to the doctor on a regular basis
14.) Did your doctor discuss male menopause at any of your visits?
    A.) Yes
    B.) No
15.) Did you ask your physician about male menopause?
    A.) Yes
    B.) No
16.) Is your physician male or female?
    A.) Male
    B.) Female
17.) Are you more likely to inquire about male menopause at your next doctor's visit?
    A.) Yes
    B.) No
18.) If you answered "No" to Question #17, why not? Please briefly explain:

_____
_____

19.) After completing this questionnaire, do you feel you know what questions to ask your physician?
    A.) Yes
    B.) No

*Thank you for your time in completing this very important questionnaire.

This questionnaire has been adapted from research literature by leading authors on the topic of male menopause. The majority of the questions are based on Jed Diamond's research, which can be retrieved from http://www.menalive.com.

APPENDIX D
Posttest

INSTRUCTIONS: Please select only one response per question!

Do I Have Andropause?   http://www.andropause.com/diagnosis/quiz.asp

Andropause

Getting Old is Natural. Feeling Old is Optional.

| About Andropause | Diagnosis | Treatment Options | About Andriol | Talking to Your Doctor | FAQs | Patient Resources |

Do I Have Andropause?

Diagnosis

Do I Have
Andropause?
Take our Quiz to find
out...

Do I Have Andropause?

Andropause is a hormone-related condition of
low-testosterone. It usually occurs in males aged 40 and
onwards. Take this test and find out if you have the
symptoms of andropause.

To complete the quiz, simply fill in the answers by clicking
on a "YES" or "NO" box. Once you have finished, click "Submit"
to view your results.

**Don't forget to answer all the questions to view
your results.**

	YES	NO
1. Do you have a decrease in strength and/or endurance?	○	○
2. Do you have a lack of energy?	○	○
3. Do you have a decrease in your sex drive (libido)?	○	○
4. Are you more sad and/or grumpy than usual?	○	○
5. Have you lost height?	○	○
6. Have you noticed a decreased enjoyment in life?	○	○
7. Have you noticed a recent deterioration in your ability to play sports?	○	○
8. Has there been a recent deterioration in your work performance?	○	○
9. Are your erections less strong?	○	○
10. Are you falling asleep after dinner?	○	○

Read carefully, did/does any of the following apply to you?

Current age:

_____

Note: This copy does not represent the actual size of the original test.

Next Section >>

Contact Us | Site Map | Privacy Policy | Terms of Usr
© 2002 NV Organon. All rights reserved.

APPENDIX E

QUESTIONNAIRE (PRETEST) RESULTS

Question No.	A Yes	B No	C	D	E	F	Totals	Question No.	%A	%B	%C	%D	%E	%F
#1	47	57					104	#1	45.2%	54.8%	0.0%	0.0%	0.0%	0.0%
#2	35	14	55				104	#2	33.7%	13.5%	52.9%	0.0%	0.0%	0.0%
#3	3	27	57	17			104	#3	2.9%	26.0%	54.8%	16.3%	0.0%	0.0%
#4	17	15	72				104	#4	16.3%	14.4%	69.2%	0.0%	0.0%	0.0%
#5	4	6	13	15		66	104	#5	3.8%	5.8%	12.5%	14.4%	0.0%	63.5%
#6	2	39	10	53			104	#6	1.9%	37.5%	9.6%	51.0%	0.0%	0.0%
#7	74	29				1	104	#7	71.2%	27.9%	0.0%	0.0%	0.0%	1.0%
#8	28	7	16	28	24	1	104	#8	26.9%	6.7%	15.4%	26.9%	23.1%	1.0%
#9	3	71	29			1	104	#9	2.9%	68.3%	27.9%	0.0%	0.0%	1.0%
#10	37	24	4	38		1	104	#10	35.6%	23.1%	3.8%	36.5%	0.0%	1.0%
#11	9	88		1		6	104	#11	8.7%	84.6%	0.0%	1.0%	0.0%	5.8%
#12	1	2	2	93	0	6	104	#12	1.0%	1.9%	1.9%	100.0%	0.0%	5.8%
#13	54	28	10	5		7	104	#13	51.9%	26.9%	9.6%	4.8%	0.0%	6.7%
#14	4	94				6	104	#14	3.8%	90.4%	0.0%	0.0%	0.0%	5.8%
#15	4	92				8	104	#15	3.8%	88.5%	0.0%	0.0%	0.0%	7.7%
#16	84	14				6	104	#16	80.8%	13.5%	0.0%	0.0%	0.0%	5.8%
#17	61	37				6	104	#17	58.7%	35.6%	0.0%	0.0%	0.0%	5.8%
#18	76	28					104	#18	73.1%	26.9%	0.0%	0.0%	0.0%	0.0%
#19	76	22				6	104	#19	73.1%	21.2%	0.0%	0.0%	0.0%	5.8%

APPENDIX F

QUESTIONNAIRE (POSTTEST) RESULTS

Question No.	A Yes	B No	C No responses	Totals	Question No.	%A	%B	%C
#1	26	65		91	#1	28.6%	71.4%	0.00%
#2	27	64		91	#2	29.7%	70.3%	0.00%
#3	29	59	3	91	#3	31.9%	64.8%	3.30%
#4	16	75		91	#4	17.6%	82.4%	0.00%
#5	6	85		91	#5	6.6%	93.4%	0.00%
#6	9	78	4	91	#6	9.9%	85.7%	4.40%
#7	30	61		91	#7	33.0%	67.0%	0.00%
#8	11	79	1	91	#8	12.1%	86.8%	1.10%
#9	32	59		91	#9	35.2%	64.8%	0.00%
#10	22	69		91	#10	24.2%	75.8%	0.00%
#11					#11			

Note:

No. 11 reflects the age of the respondents

There were 104 surveys distributed; and 13 men chose not to do the posttest